Amy Lane is the host of iTunes-featured running podcast *Well Far* (which has had more than 250k downloads) and Digital Editor of *Women's Health* UK. She is a qualified fitness expert and regarded as one of the most influential editors in health and wellness.

When not podcasting or editing, Amy regularly speaks at health and fitness events and can be found sharing insights into healthy living via Instagram. You can find her at @Wellness_Ed.

She has been featured by *The Telegraph*, *Get The Gloss*, *Elle*, *PopSugar*, *The Times* and *Esquire* and is passionate about inspiring women everywhere to fall in love with fitness for mental and physical boons.

Amy lives in London with her husband Ted.

To Kate, for helping her son find his path in life and in doing so, helping me to find mine. You're with us every step of the way.

I Can Run

AN EMPOWERING GUIDE TO RUNNING WELL FAR

AMY LANE

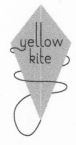

First published in Great Britain in 2020 by Yellow Kite
An imprint of Hodder & Stoughton
An Hachette UK company

1

Copyright © Amy Lane 2020

A CIP catalogue record for this title is available from the British Library

Trade Paperback ISBN 978 1 529 34348 9
eBook ISBN 978 1 529 36574 0

Typeset in Celeste by Palimpsest Book Production Ltd, Falkirk, Stirlingshire

Printed and bound in Great Britain by Clays Ltd, Elcograf S.p.A.

Hodder & Stoughton policy is to use papers that are natural, renewable
and recyclable products and made from wood grown in sustainable forests.
The logging and manufacturing processes are expected to conform
to the environmental regulations of the country of origin.

Yellow Kite
Hodder & Stoughton Ltd
Carmelite House
50 Victoria Embankment
London EC4Y 0DZ

www.yellowkitebooks.co.uk

Contents

INTRODUCTION:
Going Well Far 1

CHAPTER 1:
Your First Steps To Greatness 11

CHAPTER 2:
Finding Your Tribe 51

CHAPTER 3:
Now You're Up And Running 68

CHAPTER 4:
Food For Thought 87

CHAPTER 5:
Weights Off Your Mind 122

CHAPTER 6:
The Art Of Doing F*ck All 145

CHAPTER 7:
Let's Call It A Comeback 175

CHAPTER 8:
Girl Bossing It 192

CHAPTER 9:
Thinking On Your Feet 217

CHAPTER 10:
See You At The Start Line 243

Epilogue 263
Training Plans 265
Your Little Black Book Of Running 279
Acknowledgements 290
Resources 292
References 296

Going Well Far

Whoever said you can't run away from your problems was wrong. Millions will tell you that running helped them to get over a trauma, be that a break-up or a bereavement. Or deal with deep-rooted mental-health problems. And though I don't personally think you ever *get over* those blows in life – I think you simply learn to accept them – running was the self-help mechanism that saved me.

A morning 5k or a 10-minute breeze around the block at lunch has become an exercise-shaped painkiller for the travails of life. Running helps me to pause the negative thought loop when I. Just. Can't. Stop. Replaying. *THAT EMAIL* over in my head. It gives my mind something else to obsess over – though normally that's simply replaying 'how much further?!'

But it's much more than a distraction. Running has taught me that I'm enough. It's taught me that I don't have to prove myself through fat percentages or body shape, and that I can run a race for the joy that's in it, not just the finish time.

My journey to marathon running was not linear, however. There's no straight line from school cross country, to Parkrun, to race day. In fact, if you had to draw it, it would most likely resemble a three-year-old's drawing proudly displayed on the fridge – all squiggly lines with no sense of direction. Crucially, though, all those squiggles have helped me to make sense of my life out of running trainers. Before running set my mind in the right direction, I admit, I was a mess.

This came to a head a few years into my job as the digital editor of *Women's Health*, when I was offered a place in the London Marathon. In the running community this is equivalent to finding a golden ticket (a record 457,861 applicants registered for a ballot place in the 2020 Virgin Money London Marathon, and only 40,000 were successful). But when a free bib was dangled in front of me, I didn't jump and click the heels of my Adidas Boosts together like a bad stock photo – I started to laugh with panic. To me, I was not a real runner.

Yes, I jogged occasionally around the park or ran when a fitness launch or weekend away with no gym required it, but I wasn't fast like 'real runners' and I definitely wasn't one of the UK run commuters who, according to Strava,[1] clocked a total of 21.7 million kilometres to work in 2018. I wasn't even close to clocking three runs a week (the number most beginner marathon plans suggest you should be doing before dialling up the distance). But how could I say 'thanks but no thanks' to the opportunity? And more importantly, how could I say no in front of colleagues and bosses who believed that I worked hard but worked out harder?

It's a nauseating line, I know. But it's one that I'd used while desperately pitching myself during the interview process. And somehow, it worked. It's why for months I was proud of being in the office until security turned the lights off. It's why I'd then head home and crash out for a few short hours before rushing out the door again for an early-morning workout class. The idea of slowing down was incomprehensible.

I would tell friends, colleagues and my social circle, 'I only need five hours' sleep.' I left out the fact that I actually needed five hours' sleep *plus* five super-strong coffees throughout the day. The reality was that I was surviving on cortisol and caffeine.

To understand why I put so much pressure on myself, and to understand why the idea of running a marathon didn't feel like a wonderful opportunity, but instead made me clam up for fear of failure, I need to unpack some of my past for you.

As a child raised by a single mother, research suggests that I should have fared significantly worse in a number of areas, most notably emotional development and career. But when my father cut all ties with my family when I was just five years old, my mum made sure I wanted for nothing. I watched her hustle with a quiet ferocity that couldn't be stopped. She worked multiple jobs late into the night so that my sister and I had Marks & Spencer cereal and Troll Dolls just like the other kids. When she wasn't teaching aerobics to 300+ people in Swindon (yes, she was the female Joe Wicks of the 90s), she sat in front of the TV sewing 80s-style exercise belts to sell the next day to the women jumping along with her in the sports hall. She was a combination of Jane Fonda and Del Boy – a wheeler-dealer in Lycra. And so, not once did I question that I wouldn't achieve what friends from unbroken homes would achieve. I just knew that for me to do the same, I needed to hustle too. And that's exactly what I did.

After flunking my A-levels the first time around, I worked in a pub and put myself through college at 20 before moving to the capital to study at the London College of Fashion. While friends at university were paying rent using the Bank of Mum and Dad, I worked multiple jobs to cover the eye-watering cost of studying in the UK's most expensive city.

At times it was brutal. One winter I ended up in A&E because, after finishing work at 5am, tired and freezing because our East Finchley flat had holes in the roof (great as aircon in the summer, less useful during 2009's extreme snowfall) I fell asleep with a hot-water bottle in between my legs. Such was my level of exhaustion that by the time I woke up the heat from the hot-water bottle had seared third-degree burns into the insides of my knees. Had I seen a doctor right away, I would have been patched up and sent on my merry way. However, I had to work. I couldn't afford to miss any shifts, so I slapped on a couple of plasters and hustled on. Four days later I couldn't hustle any longer. In fact, I couldn't even walk. Burns can get infected easily, you see, and the A&E doctor said I was lucky to avoid sepsis. I haven't used a hot-water bottle since.

This work-first mentality stayed with me after graduation and into my first job. I treated every day like I was one step closer to proving to myself (and my waste-of-space father, should I ever see him again) that against the odds, I'd made it. However, despite my burgeoning success in the workplace, I never shook the sense that because I'd hustled so hard to get there, I wasn't worthy. I thought that it was graft, not skill, that had got me there and eventually that wouldn't be enough. I'd get found out. I felt like a career con-artist. That feeling made me try far too hard at the stuff I was good at in life, and quit the things I wasn't good at. Running was one of those things.

And so, circling back to that marathon offer, sitting on a sofa that was too small, next to my boss. For a moment, he said nothing. Perhaps he was confused as to why this supposedly fitness-obsessed woman in front of him wasn't champing at the bit to run and was actually flushing with panic. Whatever it was, I filled the silence with excuses. I told him that I simply had no time to train around my workload. I explained that the longest I'd run in months was 200m sprints on a treadmill. I said I didn't look like a marathon runner.

He sat there and listened, a little perplexed at the intensity of my excuses. To him, it really wasn't that big a deal, but for me, right then, I was verbally processing my big deal: I was scared of not being fast enough and, ultimately, good enough. In my mind real runners had spindly legs the thickness of my ankle. They ran come rain or shine, and ordered soda and lime on a Saturday night to ensure they weren't hungover for Sunday Runday. When their 5.30am alarm went off they thought, 'Let's run this!' Not, 'FFS, it's *so* early and still dark!' Real runners didn't give up after 2 miles to stumble into the nearest coffee shop and order an almond milk flat white.

And so, I had a decision to make. I could either let fear stop me from giving it a go, or I could use that sensation in the pit of my stomach to re-script the rest of my life and deal with the demons that had been hanging over me since my teens. There are no prizes for guessing which option I took, and I'm pleased to say that I've never looked back. Since then I've gone on a journey that's taken me through the streets of London, along the Thames and even across the Seine in Paris.

Over the following pages I'll share a journey that many have run before me, but here I'll also double down on how marathon running has taught me self-compassion, self-belief and self-worth. I want this book to show you that all our preconceptions about 'real runners' are wrong. Everyone is a runner. I can run and most importantly, *you* can run.

'I am a runner
when ~~I'm~~
~~lighter~~
~~when I'm~~
~~thinner~~
~~when I'm~~
~~faster~~
when I put on
my trainers'

How To Use This Book

I Can Run is as much about you as it is me. It's about getting the most out of *your* running journey, no one else's. This book is not a training manual for 'runners', it's a companion for every woman who has ever experienced the softly spoken, yet sadistic voice in her head whispering, 'you can't run'.

Over 10 chapters you will be put on a path to personal glory. Whatever your starting point and whatever your goal – you'll get there. Here's how.

STEP ONE: PARK YOUR EGO

Because this is going to be humbling and embarrassing, but also *empowering*. Confidence is a wonderful thing, and for those of you that have it in your comfort zones, the aim here will be to build it in your discomfort zones. For those of you who lack confidence in your day-to-day, the plan is to build it in running so that you can apply it to every aspect of your life.

But that confidence won't appear immediately. Running is a great leveller. No matter your age, your profession, your weight or your gender, your running journey will have highs and lows. For every new milestone there will be a time when you'll be overtaken by a 14-year-old at Parkrun. Ditching your ego will allow you to deal with these moments with zero sense of embarrassment.

So far in my own marathon journey I've accidentally spat on a stranger, narrowly missed shooting a snot rocket onto a running pal and gone nose to bar with a lamppost while trying to email and run. Yes, we runners (that's you and me, by the way) are an awkward, calamity-prone species. So, welcome to the club. These hilarious and unfiltered moments help you to better connect with your body, and with every faceplant there's an opportunity to rise up stronger.

STEP TWO: LAY STRONG FOUNDATIONS

If step one was about letting your guard down, then step two is about learning how to build yourself back up again, both mentally and physically. In addition to finding the confidence to call yourself a runner, you need to bullet-proof the body and mind that are going to carry you through all this.

First, you'll learn that 'running to get fit' is a phrase that should be buried in the graveyard of bad health advice. Instead you need to get fit to run, and that will take you from the pavement and park loop to the track, the weights room and, pleasingly, the sofa. That's because, with the support of my squad of experts, you'll understand that there's much more to running than putting one foot in front of the other. You need to eat well, you need to get strong and you need to *chill the fuck out*. If your body is going to last the course, then setting aside time to sit in front of the telly is crucial.

STEP THREE: CHASE DOWN PROGRESS

Now, this is where your journey really picks up the pace. With expert tips and learnings from my own journey, the opportunity is there to power towards your own race day. You'll be able to try the running plans that built me up to half-marathon and marathon success, and learn all the tips you need to survive start line nerves and crash through any proverbial wall. Equally, you'll learn just how quickly your running success can slide into injury and disaster if you don't practise the 10 per cent mileage rule and realise that no one ever said running was easy! It's hard and you need to look after yourself. But these pages will teach the practices that ensure you make it to race day. '

By buying this book you've already taken the first step, so now it's time to take the next one. Now's the time to let go of the beliefs that you can't do it and learn how you can. It's time to go well far.

The 'I Can Run' Mindset

- Forget times and focus on feelings
- Use social media as a companion, not a comparison
- Food is fuel and you're going to need lots of it
- Train smarter, not more
- The success of your next run starts with recovering from your last one
- Listen to your body and be OK with missing workouts when life happens
- Run for the joy that's in it and be proud of every step

CHAPTER 1

Your First Steps to Greatness

My Journey

Throughout this book I'll be sharing my own experiences, running alongside expert explainers and a collection of inspirational stories from real runners. Here, as ever, it makes sense to start at the beginning. Becoming a runner should be as easy as lacing up your trainers and getting outside. Sadly, for so many women that doesn't feel like the case. We're under-represented on start lines and all too often are the victims of negative self-talk that keeps us from moving forward. I was no different. But it only took my first steps to realise that I had it wrong all along. From timid novice to confident marathon runner, during my own journey I've met and read about people who prove that everyone is a runner, and these are the tools to help you prove it . . .

'I think I may have just sharted.' These were the first seven words that came out of my mouth as I crossed the London Marathon finish line. Quickly followed by my vomiting into a sick bag and a short stint in the St John Ambulance tent. After precisely 3 hours and 59 minutes of running, that's how my body decided to reward me.

You may think it wasn't my finest moment, but I'd disagree. When you've strived for something so hard, you'll go to any lengths to make it happen and that includes a nauseating sprint finish. Plus, any shame from spewing in public was quickly forgotten about when the medal with its royal red ribbon was placed around my neck. To me, this medal meant more than marathon memorabilia; it was confirmation that I'd kicked my self-doubt to the kerb. And in front of 750,000 spectators, no less.

In my mind, I was now officially a runner. But it also made me realise how wrong I was to wait so long before awarding myself that title. I'd actually been a runner for a long time. I'd been a runner since a friend asked me, 'What did you do this weekend?' And I told them about my first Parkrun. I'd been a runner since I got new trainers and spent 10 minutes trying to get the best Instagram shot of them. I'd been a runner since I went on a jog around the block to burn off the day's office-related anxiety. But self-doubt is a pernicious thing and it has no qualms about lying to you.

Globally, female participation in marathon running is growing. Yet here in the UK, there remains a substantial divide in the number of men and women who sign up for the challenge. According to the world's largest marathon study,[2] only 36 per cent of British marathon runners are female, which means nearly twice as many men toe the start line.

A year after running the London Marathon I crossed the Channel Tunnel to do the same on French soil. In Paris, the number of female finishers is fewer than the UK – only 27 per cent of their 60,000 race runners are women. And the disparity was unpleasantly obvious. On the Eurostar a friend whispered in my ear, warning: 'The start pens are full of guys and because there aren't enough portaloos, some runners adopt a festival mentality and discreetly whip it out before letting things flow.' Essentially it was a heads-up to be careful of guys weeing up the back of my Lululemons. And though I avoided the splash zone, after spending 90 minutes crammed into the starting pen, I couldn't help but feel outnumbered.

At times on the course, I battled to keep my share of the road as men whizzed by, elbows out. Some even had their arms spread at right angles to protect *their* precious running spot. Once, I failed to look over my shoulder before overtaking another runner and received a condescending, 'Hey missy, this is my lane,' and a jab to the ribs.

Paris lacked the carnival atmosphere of London but the competitive nature and speed actually served me well. I slashed minutes from my previous marathon time. However, three-and-a-bit hours stuck in the thick of it made me think: marathon running still doesn't feel truly inclusive.

The fight to establish women's long-distance racing isn't new. It has been a running battle for more than 50 years. In 1967 Kathrine Switzer made headlines at the Boston Marathon because, at the time, this was a men-only race. Switzer had managed to pull the proverbial wool over race officials' eyes by not using her first name on the entry form and avoiding the obligatory pre-race medical by sending in her coach with a health certificate instead. It worked. She made it to the start line undetected and it wasn't until 2 miles into the race that officials realised she had a vagina. By that point, it was too late. She was running, and despite their best efforts to pull her off the course, they couldn't.

Switzer's run made ripples around the world, but they quickly faded. Five years later, in the 70s, women were still striving for equality within sport. The Amateur Athletic Union – America's governing body for marathons – did grant women permission to enter races, but with one caveat: they had to start 10 minutes before or after male runners, or from a different start pen altogether. The six women running the 1972 New York Marathon didn't agree. So as the starting gun fired to start the women's race, they sat down. And there they stayed until it was time for the men to get going.

Today, the rules separating sexes only apply at elite level. It's now merely a requirement that affords professional runners the opportunity to qualify for world-record-time attempts. But, if gender segregation is no longer a thing, and race running is a sport that welcomes everyone, then why does the gender play gap still exist for everyday athletes? One rationale I subscribe to is that, until recently, the stereotype of a runner hasn't been one that many women connect with. At its most basic, too many women have been led to believe that running means skinny, and that to be part of the club, you have to look the part.

How wrong they are.

WHAT DOES A RUNNER LOOK LIKE?

It's true that elite runners are often thin, muscular and gangly individuals photographed in tiny tops and micro pants. But they are the 1 per cent, and though they take pride of place in advertising campaigns, they aren't representative of the sweat-soaked majority running in all shapes, sizes, skin colours and ages.

I like to think of it in simple terms. If you run and have a body, then you have a runner's body.

That's not to be blasé, either. The single-mindedness of my definition is a new discovery for me, too. I fell victim to the runner's body myth in secondary school, when more often than not, the skinnier the runner the faster their cross-country time. But, today, the relationship between size and speed isn't as simple as you'd think.

At the 2018 London Marathon, British long-distance runner Charlotte Purdue challenged the perception of an elite runner's body. Previously, Purdue had been accused of being 'too strong to be a marathon runner' by those supposedly in the know. But on that day, she ran the race of her life and clocked the third-fastest London Marathon time by a British woman. She also knocked nearly four minutes off her PB (personal best). Essentially, Purdue muscled her way into the history books and proved that body image cannot predict race results.

As I am writing this, a woman in America is waiting for official confirmation from Guinness World Records that at 24 stone and 7 pounds she is the heaviest woman to have completed a marathon. And she's just one of many runners who, in her own words, was told she was 'too fat to run'. The truth is, yes, bodyweight increases the load of running and some medical professionals will caution against the extra stress on the heart; however, the story that size is entirely insurmountable is outdated.

There are plenty more women who challenge the perception of what a runner looks like. Captained by mental-health advocates Bryony Gordon and Jada Sezer, 700 women ran a 10k in their underwear in 2018 in London. Their goal? To celebrate women's bodies and boost the confidence of women of all ages, shapes and sizes.

And it's not just in races where the image of what a runner looks like is being challenged. Last year, somebody somewhere became the 5,000,000th person to run Parkrun. But what's more interesting than the number of runners is the average Parkrun completion time: today, it's nearly 7 minutes slower than it was when the event began. This shows that the world-famous 5k is now attended by runners of all abilities; and by the simple law of averages, 5 million runners means thousands of different body types have taken on the run and won.

When researching this book I stumbled upon the story of Maggie Nolting, who had just added more than 90 minutes to her half-marathon PB. This might not sound like something to shout about, that is until you discover that Nolting completed the most recent race entirely on crutches. She had fractured her foot and been told by doctors that as long as she didn't put any weight on it she could keep exercising. Racing on crutches was her workaround.

And Nolting isn't the only one to defy odds in making it over the finish line. Since 2015 an eye surgeon named Dr Vivienne Hau has been helping visually impaired runners to race at speeds that many runners with full sight would love to clock.

Closer to home, Claire Lomas made history, competing as the 'bionic woman'. In 2012, despite being a paraplegic, Lomas started the London Marathon with the 36,000 other participants. She walked a few miles a day for 17 days to finish the course using a bionic ReWalk robotic exoskeleton, which relies on motion sensors to help her move and lift her legs. Since then, she has gone on to finish many more races, including a half marathon while 16 weeks pregnant.

Running, you see, really is for everyone.

HOW TO FINALLY FEEL LIKE A RUNNER

Overcoming internal voices that tell us we can't do something is a battle that running helped me win. But first, I had to stock my arsenal with strategies that would finally get me out of the starting blocks for good. Consider these your kickstart.

1. Training for life not the finish line

Think about it like this: race day is just one of the 70(ish) runs you'll do over a 16-week training plan. The distance is less than 10 per cent of the total miles you've already run before race day. And so there's no obligation to put pressure on crossing the finish line in record time. Instead you should take pride in the journey as a whole. As new runners, I think you can benefit far more from running to feel happy/proud/grateful (circle as appropriate) rather than chasing down a time to validate your efforts. I feel we should place equal value on every run that we show up for, not just the ones with chip times.

2. Know why running is worth it

To outsmart the excuses and mental hurdles that plague all runners (yes, not just you) like, *I'm too tired, I need to work through lunch* and *I don't have time*, it helps to know why running is beneficial beyond calorie burn. There are plenty more boons to running that I believe need more airtime. Let me walk you through my favourites:

- **Youthful mind**
  Running can't turn back time but it can help to keep you in the moment mentally. Research in *Psychonomic Review*[3] found that regular exercise helps combat age-related mental decline. Getting to 70 and still feeling 55? I'll take that.

- **Lifestyle medicine**
  Regular running can help to counter the ill effects of modern sedentary lifestyles by up to 40 per cent. The research published in *Progress in Cardiovascular Disease*[4] found that runners live approximately three years longer than non-runners.

- **Happier working week**
  Various studies have concluded that regular cardio can help combat the stress[5] and strain of the daily grind. The good news is, your runs needn't be as long as 60-minute gym sessions either. Just half an hour is enough to boost sleep, mood and concentration.

- **Healthier sex life**
  A study published in *Archives Of Sexual Behavior*[6] found that one hour of exercise four days a week over nine months is all it takes to have better sex, more often. Let's call this active recovery.

- **Boost joint and bone health**
  While it's true that running can cause niggly knees for some, it's not true for all. David Felson, a researcher and epidemiologist at Boston University School of Medicine, discovered that if you're healthy with no history of injuries, running at a pace of 8–10-minute miles can be beneficial for joints[7].

3. Set realistic goals to remove fear

I'll admit it: choosing a marathon was a lofty goal for an aspiring runner – after all, it's thought that just 1 per cent of the world's population have completed this distance. However, when you break the big goal down into manageable chunks it gives the body a chance to prepare while also getting your mind used to success. It sounds obvious, and that's because it is, but a step-by-step guide to get from A to B is far easier than getting there in one giant leap.

For example: 'I'm going to run an organised 5k this week because it's an official race and a distance I know I'm fit enough to run.' It'll be a stepping stone towards your larger goal. By doing this, you get the chance to practise race prep and running in big groups, enjoy the taste of success and then move on to the next micro goal with a medal in the bag.

4. Thinking a failed run is the end

Success is not final, failure is not fatal: it is the courage to continue that counts.

— Winston Churchill

OK, Churchill's not the classic choice to paste across a sunset and slap on Instagram as an inspirational meme, but these words ring true. People tell you to learn from your mistakes but that's a hard pill to swallow when you're on the sofa with a bag of peas on your throbbing shin splints. However, it's these downfalls that often give you the time to breathe and get feedback from your mis-steps. Just because you got injured once it doesn't mean you will again, if you take the right steps to prevent it. Every run is an opportunity to learn from others and about yourself.

HOW TO START RUNNING

If you want to make running your healthy habit that sticks, you need to fit running into your lifestyle rather than trying to shoehorn your lifestyle into a running plan. Too often I've seen friends and colleagues who are either brand new to running, or attempting a running rebirth, sign up to a race and subsequently try to change all aspects of their daily grind in one week to achieve it; new morning run routines, new nutrition plan, a new weekend schedule set around a long run or a new weekly yoga class. Diving into all this change without any thought of personalisation can set you on the path to failure.

First off, if you know getting up at the last possible moment works best for you, why change it? Just because other runners get their miles in before breakfast doesn't mean you have to. There are 24 hours in a day and – work aside – you're in charge of your schedule. Equally, if you do bounce out of bed like an African springbok, then lay out your kit the night before and crush your morning cardio.

Still not sure? Ask yourself these questions to find out what will work for you:
When the alarm goes off are you . . .?
a) Up and at 'em
b) A snooze-three-times kind of person
c) Effed off that it's morning already

It's 8.30am. Are you . . .?
a) One hour into your work day
b) Arriving at work with a coffee in hand
c) Running around the house looking for your keys

When it comes to breakfast do you . . .?
a) Eat it at work at 9am
b) Put it off until 11am as you're not hungry
c) Can't function until you've eaten it

The work facilities are . . .?

a) A microwave and instant coffee

b) On-site showers that you'd go barefoot in

c) One shower that you'd only brave in flip-flops

Your idea of the perfect lunch hour is . . .?

a) An hour of catching up on life admin using work internet

b) Getting outside and away from technology

c) Working through so you can leave early #flexitime

Coffee gets you fired up for a run, but . . .?

a) You daren't have it after 3pm or you'll be awake at midnight

b) You need to eat or it gives you a dodgy stomach

c) There are no buts. You can have it anytime and still sleep

You'd describe your workday as . . .?

a) Uneventful

b) Manageable when you take screen breaks

c) Hectic and often plays on your mind

It's 7pm and you've just got through the door. Now you need to . . .?

a) Cook dinner because no one else will

b) Throw something together before doing more work

c) Microwave the home-cooked meal you batch-cooked last Sunday

At 9pm more often than not you are . . .?

a) Laying out your clothes for the next day

b) Snuggled up on the sofa with a BBC One thriller

c) Scrolling social media

Before going to sleep you . . .?
a) Leave yourself a motivational note next to your alarm
b) Check in with work pals about tomorrow's run
c) Count down the hours until you have to wake up again

Every year you look forward to summer because:
a) No more coats
b) You hate running in the dark
c) Longer evenings to spend time outside

As – Get it done first thing
If you answered mostly As then you're a morning person in training. Tap into your lark tendencies and reap the rewards of running in the morning, which include pushing your metabolism to burn more calories, cooler temperatures in summer and better sleep at night. But just because you're raring to go it doesn't mean your body always is. As you sip your morning coffee, work through a mobility and activation routine. Then both your mind and body will be in sync and ready to run.

Bs – Enjoy a midday runbreak
Your mostly B choices are indicative of your balanced approach to work–life. You're organised and a dependable employee; however, you know that chewing on a Pret sandwich over emails isn't what your mind needs at midday. Lunch breaks equate to 30 extra days (or six weeks) of annual leave, so take them. That hour holds the potential for an extra 25k of running over the week, with time left over for a quick wash in the office showers. Just don't forget to set off bang on 12 while your energy stores are still stocked from your breakfast. Later than that and you risk running on empty.

Cs – Round off the day with a run

I have one word for you: runmute. Your choice of mostly C highlights your need to end the day on a high – a runner's high to be precise. Which is good news considering the growing body of research[8] to support the theory that the human body performs best between 4 and 7pm when your core temperature peaks. If you're in training for a PB, now is the best time for an interval session – your endurance, strength, aerobic capacity and reaction time are all operating at full throttle.

---

3 tips to stop you cancelling morning runs:

- Put your kit on the radiator the night before. Then at 6am you can look forward to a warm Lycra hug waiting for you.

- If you can't function until you have coffee but are short on time in the AM, fill up a Thermos the night before and put it on your nightstand. Many insulated flasks will keep hot drinks warm for 12 hours – far longer than you'll sleep, I bet.

- Invest in a wake-up light so you have a personal sunrise whatever time you wake up. These clocks have changed my mornings.

'All toenails go to heaven'

Follow The Leader

To get your new-found enthusiasm for running off on the right foot, meet Emma Kirk-Odunubi. She is a footwear expert and sports scientist who has been in the running industry for over 10 years. Day-to-day she works with a variety of sports men and women, from novice runners to elite athletes. Emma is a running biomechanics nerd who matches the perfect footwear to the individual runner, and takes pride in being known as the trainer geek. This places her in a prime position to share all her thinking on your feet, which can empower you to be the best runner possible. Over to Emma for her comprehensive guide.

PUTTING YOUR FOOT DOWN

There are nearly 7 million people participating in running in England alone, according to a Statista survey.[9] All of them had to start somewhere. Most of them will have started with the same first thought: I need a new pair of trainers. But they, and you, need to slow down.

Firstly, you need to learn how you run and what your feet do when you run. To do this you need a gait analysis.

WHAT IS A GAIT ANALYSIS?

This is the way of understanding which shoes suit your stride. Head to an independent retailer who is unbiased on brand selection and who will help you to get the best shoe based on how you move, what'll fit your foot and what you can afford.

It sounds simple and that's because it is. The expert at the shop will ask you to hop on a treadmill and walk or run for a bit. They'll watch you and watch your feet. The benefit? If you're new to running this takes the stress out of what is a very important decision. The problem today, with the rise of online shopping, is that a lot of people buy trainers based on guesswork or, more likely, how they look. And, sure, looking and feeling the part out on the road helps, but what's infinitely better is to have a shoe that looks cool and also has the seal of approval from someone who is an experienced runner and is trained to give fitting advice.

I do understand, however, that while passing the buck to an expert can be freeing, it can also be disconcerting. Especially when new shoes often end up as a significant outlay. It can therefore help mentally to have a grasp of what's going on. Runners want information and data, and so I'm going to try and explain a little about gait analysis and footwear selection. For the running geeks among you, get ready for a white-knuckle ride of nerding out . . .

Pronation

To start with, I have to cover a word bandied about in the industry so much that many don't truly understand its meaning. Pronation. There is a huge misconception that this is bad. In fact, it is a natural movement where the foot rolls inwards with each stride, and 99 per cent of feet do it to help your body absorb the shock from the ground.

Pronation, when excessive, is deemed a negative by some because it begins to alter mechanics further up your body, such as in the knees and hips. In truth, research has never labelled pronation as the sole cause of injury, though that hasn't stopped much of the footwear industry always selling shoes with support, stating that it's needed to prevent over-pronation.

The makeup of your ankles and feet can cause your feet to be naturally pronated. It's where the arch of your foot folds into the floor, and is what lots of people refer to as being flat-footed. But this is no guarantee that your foot is going to overpronate when you start running. Which is why experts analyse your gait (how your foot moves through each stride) rather than simply analysing the look of your foot when you're stationary.

There are two more categories of feet beyond pronated.

Neutral

A neutral foot is one that pronates to make initial contact with the ground during each stride and absorb shock. However, after the foot is fully on the floor it doesn't continue to pronate further as your foot completes the stride (or gait cycle, if you want to sound fancy).

Supinated

A supinated foot (sometimes called underpronation) is limited in its ability to shock absorb. This foot is usually more rigid through its arch and will instead shift weight to the outside of the foot. Only a very small percentage of people have supinated feet.

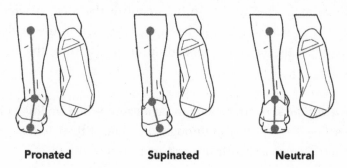

| Pronated | Supinated | Neutral |

THE SELECTION PROCESS

When it comes to footwear selection, we're not really bothered by the angle of the foot in a standing position or how the arches look in that position, either. Surprisingly for some, arch height is not a pre-determinant for the level of support you need. A high arch doesn't necessarily mean the foot is neutral and won't pronate, neither does a low arch or flat foot definitely mean a foot will overpronate.

We care about the movement through the running stride and how the ankle joint moves in relation to the knee and hip joints during that stride pattern. That is the goal of a gait analysis. And once an expert has checked you out, then they're equipped to properly upgrade your foot locker.

Types of trainers
There are different types of shoe to suit different gaits.

Supportive shoes: a foot that pronates excessively and therefore stresses your knees will usually benefit from a more supportive shoe. A supportive shoe is one that's traditionally made up of two densities of foam. One softer to help shock absorb at initial contact, plus a firmer, denser foam (also known as a shoe's post) to help control the area in which the foot pronates. This can be in the rear foot on the medial side or in the midfoot, depending on how strong the shoe is.

Neutral shoes: neutral shoes are more simple and traditionally have one density of foam throughout. Some of these foams can be soft; some can be firmer and more responsive.

The easiest way to describe footwear choice is that they all exist along a continuum. In this way you can understand that trainers don't simply sit in one category or another. As the technology and designs have advanced, shoes can vary depending on where the foot needs support or softness. It is also important to remember that footwear can be classified as more or less supportive depending on more than its foam type; the upper, which holds the foot in place, is another major determining factor.

My example continuum is designed to help you visualise where certain models sit. Understand that there can be firmer support shoes, softer support shoes, firmer neutral shoes and softer neutral shoes, which all vary in shape and function.

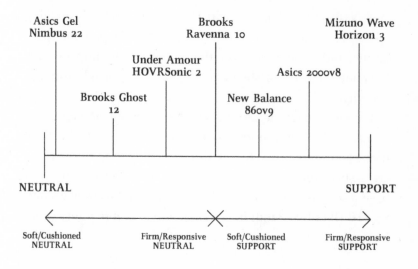

DROP THE SUBJECT

The variations don't stop with gait type, however. Drop height is another important variation and is the difference between the height of cushioning in the heel and the height in the forefoot. For example, a shoe with a drop of 4mm will have, say, 24mm of cushioning in the heel and 20mm in the forefoot. Simply put, the higher the drop of the shoe, the less stress there is on your calf muscles to work as hard.

If you have any history of calf issues or Achilles problems, be cautious in your shoe choice when it comes to drop height. I'm not saying you can't use low drop or barefoot running shoes, but consider easing yourself into them or only using them for shorter distances. Using a higher drop shoe for longer mileage will help protect your calves and Achilles from injury.

In all, it's a lot to consider, but a little knowledge can go a long way – chiefly, stopping you from glazing over when the store assistant is trying to help. Or, more importantly, helping you to read and make sense of descriptions when shopping online, rather than rely on the colourway to inform your selection, and pick a shoe that can carry you safely through training.

Incorrect footwear can throw your body out of alignment. Imagine a foot that supinates, impacting on the outside of the foot, going into a shoe that is firm and supported through the arch. This support will increase the rate the foot rolls out and have a serious effect on your knees. It'll be a breeding ground for ITB (Iliotibial Band) irritation and many more injury problems.

RUNNING SHOE GLOSSARY

This A–Z of running shoe lingo will ensure you keep a clear head when considering any new additions to your foot locker.

Cushioning: This provides comfort and shock absorption.

Eyelets: The holes that laces poke through and can be used to help create a custom fit.

Drop: The difference between the height of the heel and the height of the toe.

Footbridge: A reinforced platform under the arch between the heel and the sole that prevents the shoe from bending in the middle.

Forefoot: The inside of the shoe where the ball of your foot and toes sit.

Flat-footed: A foot that doesn't have a high arch.

Flex: How bendy the shoe is.

Flex grooves: The cuts in the tread to allow the shoe to bend.

Forefoot striker: A runner who lands on their forefoot with every stride.

Heel collar: The part of the shoe that fits around your ankle.

Heel counter: The part of the shoe that cradles the heel and helps align the foot as it strikes the ground.

Heel striker: A runner who lands on their heel first with every stride.

Insole: Material shaped like the bottom of your foot and that sits inside the shoe.

Lateral: The side of the shoe that faces outwards.

Light stability: A little bit of stability when you run.

Maximal: The most cushioned shoes out there.

Medial: The side of the shoe that faces your opposite foot.

Midsole: The part of the shoe designed to provide cushioning and shock absorption.

Midfoot striker: A runner who lands on their midfoot with every step.

Minimal: A shoe that's not got much in the way of cushioning or structure. As close to barefoot running without going shoeless.

Neutral: Shoes that don't correct pronation or supination.

Outsole: The part of the shoe that touches the ground.

Overlay: Anything that is stitched or bonded to the upper.

Pronation: When your feet roll inwards.

Sockliner: Removable foam footbeds to cover the seams and gaps in a shoe's construction.

Stack height: How high off the ground your foot is; this is related to drop.

Stability: The term given to shoes that aim to correct pronation or supination.

Supination: When your foot rolls outwards towards the lateral side of the shoe.

Toe bumper: Additional rubber on the front of a trail shoe for extra protection.

Tongue: The material in the middle of the shoe that sits between the laces and your foot. It should be pulled up tight and lined up straight between the eyestays, which anchor the eyelets.

Torsional rigidity: How little a shoe bends when twisted.

Trail shoes: Trainers designed for muddy, uneven terrain.

Tread: The rubber on the outsole.

Upper: The top part of a shoe that encases your foot.

Vamp: A part of the upper that surrounds the toebox. If you can pinch a quarter of an inch, the vamp is too baggy. If you can't wiggle your toes, it's too tight.

Volume fit: How snug or loose the shoe feels around your foot. Nothing to do with length of the shoe.

Zero drop: When the heel and forefoot height are the same. Normally seen on 'barefoot'-style shoes.

GO TO YOUR HAPPY LACE

Once you have the right shoe that fits your mechanics, lacing can further customise your fit. Try these geek tweaks on for size.

High arch/instep

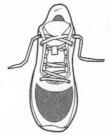

For high-arched feet, pressure can sometimes arise on the top of the foot, causing irritation, pain and even be a cause for numbing further down the foot. By creating a window of space in the affected area you can still properly secure the foot while reducing the isolated pressure point.

Wide foot

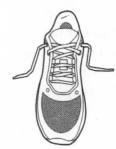

By re-lacing your trainers and missing out the first eyelets, you allow the area around the toe joints more space and less restriction. This lacing may also help those with bunions or who suffer from foot numbness.

1st heel lock lacing

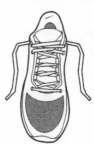

This version is the simplest in order to help with heel retention in the shoe. All trainers, once you have laced them up, have an extra eyelet hole. This eyelet is rarely used but should be. By simply lacing back through this hole you are able to better secure your foot in the shoe.

2nd heel lock lacing

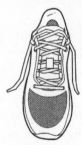

In this method for heel retention, there are loops created in the last hole of the lace system. This enables an even greater lock of the foot and ankle. This may not be for everyone as it can occasionally cause increased pressure on top of your foot, but give both options a go and work out which one works best for your foot shape.

PUNCTURE REPAIR KIT

New shoes, although an excellent first step on your journey, aren't without their pitfalls. The most wincingly obvious are blisters. The cause of blisters is sheer stress between the layers of the skin. Friction stops the skin moving while the skeletal structures underneath continue to move freely. Over time this causes your feet to heat up, damages the cellular makeup of your skin's outer layers and causes them to split. Fluid then fills the gap and creates a bubble. *Et voilà*, the pesky blister is born!

Once a blister has arisen there are a few rules that you should follow depending on the type of blister you have:

Hot spot

If you are lucky, you may not have developed a blister but a hot spot, which is just an area of reddening. You'll feel this rubbing and the smart option is simply to stop, remove your sock and shoe and make sure no stone is in there aggravating you. Then, if you are able, cover the area with a preventative plaster to stop it developing into something worse.

Blister with a roof

This will more than likely be noticed post-run and the main question is, should you drain it or just cover it. If it's small, just cover it with a plaster and let it go down on its own. If the blister is a beast, you can choose to drain it. Using a sterile wipe, clean the area and then make two small holes at the ends with a sterile needle. Once the fluid is drained, stick on a clean bandage to prevent bacteria and infection.

Blister without a roof

This is essentially an open wound. Clean the area with an antiseptic wipe to remove dirt and then let the area dry out to heal. If you need to run again, cover with a protective tissue plaster then remove it as soon as possible to let it breathe post-run. If you've got the time, give the blister a few days of healing before running again and try to discern the cause.

In addition to heat and friction, moisture is a major cause of blisters, whether that's from sweat or running through puddles. But by tackling these risk factors you can decrease the likelihood of being hobbled by a blister.

1. Dry skin is likely to blister more easily because friction is going to be greater on a rough surface. To smooth the surface of your skin, use moisturiser like cocoa butter before bed.
2. Footwear can be a cause of blistering. The shape of the shoe varies from brand to brand. Some are more narrow or wide than others and this can irritate certain areas of the foot, causing increased heat and friction. Shop around.
3. Some people have baby-soft skin and will always be more prone to blistering due to having a higher amount of collagen

in their skin. There are skin-toughening solutions available from pharmacies, so try bathing your feet in them if you always seem to suffer.

4. And finally, buy the correct socks. Do not run in cotton socks. Cotton absorbs moisture. During running, your feet will sweat and your cotton socks will absorb it and then rub against your moist feet. A technical running sock will not hold on to that moisture and your foot will be less likely to blister.

As a runner, your feet are the tools of your trade. The first rules as a beginner and taking your first steps to greatness should be to look after them. Treat them right, treat them to a new pair of shoes, and they'll take you all the way.

AMY'S WARDROBE ESSENTIALS

Now you've got your trainers sorted (thanks, Emma), let's talk about the other gear that you'll need on this journey. First things first, don't Google 'running kit'. If you do, the thousands of search results you're presented with might give you heart palpitations because, *isn't running free*? While you don't *need* all this kit, there are certain items that will make running a far more comfortable endeavour.

Sports bra

When you run your boobs bounce. (Duh!) But did you know that they can move up to 14cm? In doing so, this can strain ligaments and cause a loss of elasticity. To protect your puppies, invest in a sports bra that's properly designed to handle the movement. You want your breasts to move in unison with your torso and not bounce independently of one another.

5 tips for finding the right fit:

1. *Allow for stretch*: when deciding on what size to buy, fasten the band of the bra on the loosest hook while trying it on. Then, as it ages and becomes looser, you can tighten the fit. If you can fit two fingers between your body and the band (but no more), that's the sign of a good fit.
2. *Choose wide straps*: thin spaghetti straps have the potential to dig in. Look for wide, padded straps that are adjustable.
3. *Check for coverage*: the cups need to completely cover your breasts. Wrinkles or puckering in the fabric indicate the cups are too big. If you have side-boob that means the cup is too small, or that the style of bra is the wrong cut for your breast type.
4. *Assess comfort*: does the underwiring poke or pinch? This is a sign that the style doesn't fit.
5. *Check fabrics*: running is not the time for a cotton yoga bralette. First off, you need support, but secondly, cotton will hold sweat – putting you at risk of chafing. Choose sweat-wicking synthetic fabrics.

Running leggings

Much like yoga bras don't double as running bras, leggings designed for Savasana won't fare well when soaked in sweat. You need the workhorse of your running wardrobe to be a thoroughbred and designed for purpose.

The ultimate tights ticklist:

Fabric: choose sweat-wicking fabrics so that moisture doesn't pool on your skin. This helps prevent chills and chafe. In the summer look for Lycra with SPF to protect against harmful rays.

Drawstring: this is essential for a secure fit. No one wants to have to hoist up their tights every five strides on a run.

Pockets: you might like the idea of running out of the house with nothing more than optimism and your headphones, but when it comes down to it, that's rarely practical. Deep side pockets on leggings are essential for carrying your phone, a running gel and house keys. Once I even managed to stuff a doughnut in mine on the return leg of a 15-miler.

Zip pocket: you might wonder why you'd need this *and* deep side pockets. But you do. A zip pocket is the best place to stow a bank card. These are so light that they can accidentally fly out without you noticing as you reach for your running gel. Trust me, I've been there.

Reflective strips: running in daylight isn't always possible. Whether it's early-morning miles or runmutes in the dark, it's important to stay visible. Choose tights that have reflective detailing on the back or your legs.

Length: if you're under 5'5", shop leggings labelled as 7/8s – the slightly shorter length. There's nothing worse than tights bunching at the ankle, gathering moisture and causing a sweat rash.

Tip: sidestep fabric softener when washing your workout gear if you want it to smell fresh. The oils in this solution can clog up fabric fibres and bacteria cling to these oils, which means you'll never quite rid yourself of the smell of speedwork.

Cycling shorts

Spoiler: they're not just for cycling. A pair of well-fitting cycling shorts with deep side pockets are handy for hot races when leggings are too much.

Running sunglasses

Come rain or shine, if you're running in the UK, you'll need a pair of sunnies. They'll either act as a sunscreen for your eyes or a windshield on rainy days.

Compression kit

The scientific jury is still out on *how* effective compression kit is for boosting your performance, but there is some research to suggest it does when worn post-session. Personally, I do away with the leggings and just wear compression socks after a long run. I also wear them on flights to stop my ankles swelling.

Running jackets

If you're a fairweather runner you'll need a jacket to prevent the British weather dampening your plans of a PB. A simple shell will provide light protection against the elements while a waterproof jacket with sealed seams will keep you covered against all conditions.

Running gloves

Keeping your hands warm and dry should be a simple task but it's one that many gloves can't quite achieve. When shopping for gloves look for breathable fabrics to avoid clammy palms; styles with 'tech touch fingers' (the stuff that allows you to work your phone screen) are brilliant when it's really cold and you don't want to remove a glove to call Mum for a catch-up.

Hydration vest

If you're going to be running for over an hour, you'll need to hydrate en route. A light, compact hydration vest is your portable water station. Some will have pockets for gels and your phone too. Whatever you choose, make sure you wash and sterilise the kit after every run so it doesn't become a breeding ground for mould, mildew and bugs that will cause a bad stomach.

HOW TO KNOW WHAT TO WEAR ON A RUN

To ensure the decision to get out and run isn't harder than it needs to be, here's a handy guide on what to wear.

SNOW	COLD & DRY	WINDY	RAINY
Long-sleeve base layer	Long-sleeve base layer	Leggings or shorts	Short-sleeve t-shirt
Gilet	Leggings	Short-sleeve t-shirt	Rain jacket
Thermal leggings		Wind shield	Leggings or shorts
Ear warmers	Sunglasses		
Gloves	Gloves	Gloves	Baseball cap

COOL	SUNNY & WARM	HOT
Long-sleeve base layer	T-shirt	Vest
Shorts	Shorts	Shorts
	Sunglasses	Sunglasses
	SPF	SPF
	Baseball cap or visor	Baseball cap or visor

On The Run With . . . Hannah Bowman

Throughout this book I'm taking the opportunity to stretch my legs and chat with a roster of inspirational people who all prove the power of running. No person fits that bill better, or serves as greater inspiration in this beginning chapter than Hannah. I saw her in a local news story and immediately got in touch. Having struggled with her weight and sense of self-worth for years she eventually reached a turning point. Through running and joining her local club she has lost a life-changing amount of weight and made a new circle of friends. She is a shining example of a woman who believed she couldn't run, but set out to prove herself wrong and now you can follow her on @fat_girl_fit_transformation. This is her success story.

AL: It sounds a bit Hollywood to say that running changed your life, but it really has. You've even had those moments of rock bottom, realisation and redemption. How did running find its way into your life?

HB: I struggled with my weight through all of my life. And I was always trying to do Slimming World and Weight Watchers. I'd do them, and lose the weight then I put it back on again.

Then my dad died, and I got even fatter. I think I was a size 26 or 28. I was eating takeaways all the time. Then we went to scatter my dad's ashes and when I look back at it, it wasn't even that hard of a walk – I just couldn't do it. It was basically my mum and my brother, and me and my dog and they were up ahead. Every ten tiny steps I had to stop because I couldn't breathe; I was out of breath, I was sweating. They were all wrapped up because it was October and it was really cold, and I was sweating, taking off layers because I was so hot. I was mortified.

When you're with your mates, they know you're a fatty and they accept you for it, but it was the pitying look that my mum and my brother gave me, and I thought this is actually really embarrassing. I finally realised carrying so much excess weight was really debilitating my life and I'm the only person who can sort this out. For the rest of that day I felt so humiliated.

Not long after, we went walking again and I had to go home; I couldn't even walk 500 metres without feeling knackered. It was quite emotional. I wasn't voicing this to my mum and my brother because I was so embarrassed about it, but it was absolutely awful. I went back and fell asleep all afternoon because I was so physically knackered. And this was normal life for me, always out of breath from just walking around and doing day-to-day stuff.

The previous January I had downloaded [the NHS's] Couch to 5K app on my phone, but I was too scared to start it. Then I thought, hang on a moment, it's October now and I haven't even tried it – it'd been on my phone for so long. I came back from being with my family – it was half-term, and I'm a teacher – and I remember lying in bed, crying, thinking, 'God, this is awful. How did I let myself to get to this?' Eventually, though, that was replaced with a moment of realisation, thinking: I can lay in bed here and be a victim, or I can get up and do something about it.

And that was it. I finally opened the app on my phone, put my tracksuit bottoms and my trainers on, went out in the rain and did it. It nearly killed me but the sense of success when I got back was fabulous. It was only week 1 on the app, which was bugger all really, but the sense of success when I got home was like, 'Shit. I can do this.' It's baby steps. It was the endorphins that made me think I've got to not be a victim, I can do this and this is my way out of it.

AL: Baby steps is so key, you're right. With a lot of those eureka moments, and trying to make a big change to your life, the temptation is to go out too quickly and make it so hard you give up . . .

HB: I've done that and all I ended up with was tendonitis. This time I did Couch to 5K on my own terms, three times a week and took the dog out. And the benefits were so wide-ranging. I get quite bad anxiety and suffer from OCD, but the activity was helping so much with everything. In the winter, I always used to get depressed and deal with seasonal affective disorder when it got dark and this year I just didn't – it felt bizarre.

And the thing is, at that time, I admit, you couldn't even really call it running. My mum and my brother would still look at me when I started, and they'd be like, 'You're not really running though, are you?' I did my first 5k a month after I'd started – it was one of the brilliant Santa Runs – and it took me like 55 minutes. But all I could think was, 'Oh my god I'm doing this'. And because I was feeling good about the exercise, I didn't want to eat crap any more. When I'm not exercising I want to eat shit. And when you exercise you just feel so good, I didn't really need to follow a diet plan because I found I was naturally just eating more healthily.

I was making sure I was making healthy choices, because I know all the diet plans back to front, inside out. And I realised I didn't have to put all these Slimming World rules in or Weight Watchers rules in, I just need to eat a healthy balanced diet. And then the weight started to drop off and my body shape really started to change.

AL: And I know that joining a running club has been instrumental in getting you hooked on keeping it up. How long did it take you to get involved?

HB: So the first of November was my first proper run, and then I thought I want to meet people, I want to join a running club. But I also thought that no one would let me join, that I'm not good enough.

I searched my local running club and it did a beginners' course, but one that didn't start until the new year. I contacted them and joined their FB page, and I put up a post saying, I want to join a beginners' course but I'm really slow and really embarrassed, does it matter? And a girl got back in touch and said, I've just done it, it doesn't matter, they're really supportive. I went along, they had Christmas drinks – I remember all the dates because it was so amazing at the time, this was the third of December.

I went so that I could recognise faces when I eventually joined the course on the fifteenth of January. People were chatting to me, they were good runners, and I began telling them what I was doing and they responded, telling me it was amazing that I could do a 5k when I was carrying around 21 stone. And I said yeah, but it takes me 55 minutes, but they just told me to put it into perspective and were so encouraging and made me believe it.

AL: That's so brilliant, you must have been sold on that club straight away?

HB: I was, I volunteered at the Festive 5, which was a race that they did, then I started the Couch to 5K plan with them on the 15 January. Even though I'd done the whole programme on my own I was starting from scratch with them and I was the slowest person, but it didn't matter. I carried on and it's been amazing.

But then I got cocky. I got carried away and I thought, 'Yeah I can do these 10ks', and I got a bloody knee injury. So now I've got patella tendonitis. So I haven't run properly for four months and I've finally gone to hospital and the doctor said this will get better – thankfully! – but I've got to do a month of exercises and then start Couch to 5K from scratch again. But that's part of it. You've got to realise and accept that you're going to have your ups and downs.

AL: Now that you have a more positive running mindset, and your relationship with food is getting more positive off the back of it, have you found it easier to eat better while injured?

HB: No. Not exercising has been really hard and I regained 10 pounds. All the exercise makes me feel like a million dollars, so I want to eat sensibly. But when I've not been exercising I just feel 'ugh'. So I've slipped back into old habits. I need the exercise to maintain it.

When I went to the doctor about my knee I thought she was going to say, 'You shouldn't be running because you're big and it's bad for your joints,' and I was so happy because she's a runner and said, 'No it's great, you should run.' I've tried so many different exercises, joined the gym, done swimming and exercise classes, but my problem is I hated it. Running is great because it's free and it's helped me to realise that I like to be outside and I'm actually excited that it's cold and wet and rainy. It's really exhilarating, I don't want to be inside. So I've just joined the gym because of my knee problem, thinking I could do some uphill on the treadmill, but I can't get my arse in there to do it because it's indoors and I can't think of anything worse.

AL: It's brilliant that you've made so much progress both physically and mentally, but can I ask how this all started? How was it that the weight crept up and you reached a position that you felt you needed to make this positive change?

HB: It all happened really slowly. It literally crept up on me. When I was younger I was always bigger, although I look back on it now and realise it wasn't that big. When I was at school, I always had puppy fat. I've always had chunky legs, too, so I always thought I was fat. My perceptions were completely skewed – when I think back now, to be a size 14 would be a dream.

Then I went to uni, drank too much lager and got up to 15 stone. I graduated at 22, and from then on, I've always battled with my weight and it just went up and up. I'd join a slimming club and I'd lose two or three stone, and then I'd put back on an extra stone when I fell off the wagon. It was constantly creeping up from a really bad relationship with food and comfort eating.

AL: I think it's so encouraging that you've now worked out that for you exercise and diet go hand-in-hand. Because people say diet is the most important thing, and in many ways it is, but if you don't feel good while you're doing it, it's also bloody difficult.

HB: Yeah, totally. I've done tracking before, but as soon as you start tracking your calories, tracking this and tracking that, then it becomes a chore, and then you feel really sad about the whole situation. What I found was when I was running I didn't need to be tracking because my body was naturally telling me what I wanted to eat and what I didn't want to eat. It's weird, but it's true. It's so much to do with the mind.

AL: You're right and in more ways than just food. You've spoken before about the sense of self-worth that came from running, can you explain that a little more?

HB: I always say I'm a fatty. I still say I'm a fatty. When I go shopping I say, 'Have you got a fat girl section?' But when you're really fat, you feel like everybody is looking at you day-to-day. Moving around, you feel like you can't fit through gaps and I got really conscious that I was starting to walk like a fat person and waddle like a fat person. It felt like shit.

I knew that it was my problem and I was the only one who could do something about it, but I didn't know how to do something about it. So then I'd just feel shit and think, 'Well I'm fat anyway, what's another takeaway going to do?' In my head I thought I'd gone past the point of no return. But running has changed all that.

AL: Do you have a goal?

HB: I have a goal to be a clothes size, more than a weight. So I'd like to be a size 14 to 16. But to do that I'm going to concentrate on setting goals in running. I'm going to start doing 5ks again once I'm over my injury, and do them well. Once I can do my 5k in half an hour, I'm going to start building my distance up again. I want to get faster before I go further because dealing with the fear of being last is awful.

I did a 10k before and I finished within the cut-off time but there were no medals left. It was awful, I was so humiliated, we all missed out on the medals and we all slogged our butts out to do it. We all just wanted to cry. We were all bigger people and we were taking longer, taking like an hour 35 minutes to do this 10k. But we got there and there were no medals left. You don't realise how much this medal meant to me. They said they'll send it in the post, but that's not the same. So I want to concentrate on keeping it shorter first and realise that I may be coming last, but I still beat myself and what I would have done a year ago.

AL: I'm impressed at how you seem to have managed to keep such a positive attitude during the injury . . .

HB: They said I'd have to rest for two months, and I panicked. Running was having such an amazing impact on my life that I didn't want to give it up. I then got used to it. And I finally went back recently and had my first session on the beginners' course again at my club. And it was horrendous but I got through it. And I realised that that was it, I could always go back and it was waiting for me whenever I was ready. I was never going to have to give up. And what's helped so much is how brilliant the people at my club, Garden City runners, are. I couldn't do it without them.

AL: And how do you feel when you're running?

HB: Before I run I feel excited, because I know I'll feel amazing afterwards. I don't dread it. Then it's weird – you start off and all I can think about is getting through the first 10 minutes. I call them the 'toxic 10'. I think, Oh my god, I'm going to die! But once I push through that it changes to, Shit, I can't believe I'm doing this! And then afterwards you just feel absolutely amazing. People told me you never feel shit after a run and it's true.

For a while I was trying to do too much too soon, so I would beat myself up if I wasn't beating my time. In a way this injury has done me a favour, because I realise I need to run for the enjoyment, do it for me and it doesn't matter if I'm a minute slower this time or a minute faster next time because ultimately I'll get there.

Right now I just want big people to realise they can do it. Even people that are not big in my eyes, but are big in their own eyes. My mum and my brother were not the best in the beginning; they had no respect for me because I had become so overweight and so fat. They thought that I wouldn't stick with what I was doing. They didn't think you could call what I was doing running. But it was for me and you've got to keep that in perspective, it's about moving forward in relation to where you were at and that's what I've done. They're totally different to me now, it's like they've suddenly got respect for me. But that's nothing compared to the new-found respect I have for myself.

Your Chapter 1 Action Plan

- Stop doubting yourself and realise that you *do* have a runner's body

- Set realistic goals to remove fear

- Make sure your new running habit fits around your schedule. Don't force it

- Get a gait analysis and choose a shoe based on more than how it looks

- Get used to failure and setbacks – this is not a linear journey to success

CHAPTER 2

Finding Your Tribe

How to find strength in numbers

My Journey

'Run girl, run. Don't give up. You're stronger than you think you are. Or, I thought you were. But wait, shit, there's another hill. This is tough. Lung-searingly tough. Oh fuck it. Do give up then. No one is watching.'

In my 20s, this is how my internal monologue went every time I set out on a weekend mission to push my mileage. Which I rarely did because this negative personal chatter would bring a perfectly normal run to an abrupt end. I wasn't in a race where there's no option but to keep pressing on, and there was no sharp-tongued personal trainer to berate me into pushing through lactic acid and heavy legs. Plus, I had no other results-hungry females in close proximity to bounce off or (more likely) refuse to be out-fitnessed by. No, it was just me and my waning willpower, out on a damp run. And so, when given the choice between lapping the park one more time to hit my target distance or calling it quits and heading home for dinner, I consistently chose the latter.

That's the thing with running – you're your own driver. You get to decide how far and how fast you run. You choose if you drop down a gear or slam your foot on the gas to make it back in time for another episode on Netflix. And, the more breathless you get, the more you and only you have to psych yourself up to keep putting one foot in front of the other.

There are few other sports that require an exercise mojo quite like this. Exercise classes, for example, are totally different. When was the last time that you decided you'd had enough mid-way through a boxing class, downed gloves and left the room? Never? Thought so. Yes, the burpees between each straight-cross combo are cause to grit your teeth, but the fear of being the one woman out of 20 who couldn't roll with the punches is enough to keep you doing One. More. Uppercut. It doesn't matter how much it hurts or how likely it is that in a minute your heart is going to burst through your chest, you don't give in.

Think about that for a bit. That class is *at least* 45 minutes long. And you make it through, every time. Yet – and I very much include myself in this category – when it comes to running the urge to stop kicks in from . . . 10 minutes? And that's on a good day.

And so, this is why running, in my mind, is tougher than other forms of fitness; there is no one to call you out or outsource your motivation to when the cramps and chafing of sweaty thighs kicks in. Running requires you to be strong-willed and have an impetus that isn't going to dissolve in the inevitable buckets of sweat. What's more: results don't happen overnight and they're preceded by tiredness and sore muscles.

Perhaps it's this physically and mentally exhausting nature of running that kept it from becoming the everyday athlete's go-to fitness booster until the 1970s. It's a fact that my inner 80s child still finds hilarious, because I can't remember a time when people didn't run. But it's true. Before the 70s, exercise advice ranged from the bland to the bonkers, and the goals were so aesthetics-driven for women that, were they published today, body-positive activists would be positively apoplectic.

Take the *Every Woman's Book of Health and Beauty* published in 1930, for example. In it, women were advised that 'long distance running, jumping, hurdling, and tug-of-war, should only be for really robust girls'. Essentially, the message is that, despite London's Violet Piercy making headlines around that time for being the first woman to run a marathon, if you had a vagina and weren't considered 'robust' then physical exertion simply wasn't suitable.

Ten years later, in the 1940s, it was a different story. Women were being encouraged to exercise, although perhaps not for the right reasons: 'Girls, it seems that after your help to win the war, you'll still have another battle on your hands, legs and other bits: the battle of the bulges!' That was how one vintage exercise video kindly put it, anyway.

The issue at hand was the fact that the nation had started to move less, yet the solutions recommended to women at the time included strapping into a Slenderizer. It's a contraption that is terrifying and hilarious in equal measure. Let me explain. The Slenderizer appears to be the cousin of the Slinky (remember those?). Only this one isn't rainbow coloured and made out of plastic, but is metal and super-sized. It's also attached to an electrical current and its sole purpose is to massage fat away. As if that's even possible.

It was another couple of decades before jogging became an exercise form of its own. Interestingly, what kicked off the craze wasn't a blockbuster movie in which the lead has a chis-elled body credited to cardio, or a celebrity dropping their new healthy habit into an interview. (Many of today's exercise trends start like this. You may remember the world bending over backwards to get into a yoga class after Geri Halliwell appeared toned and tiny 'thanks to yoga'.) Back then, however, the influencer of the moment wasn't a person but a place: the bank.

In 1963, a four-page pamphlet entitled *A Jogger's Manual* appeared in Oregon banks. In little more than 250 words it introduced the nation to 'jogging', the exercise that 'is a bit more than a walk' but not quite a run. It was written by William J. Bowerman, who at the time was famous for his coaching of the University of Oregon's world record 4-mile relay team. Today, he's more famous for being the co-founder of Nike.

As a track coach, Bowerman was constantly on a mission to discover the latest and greatest training techniques for athletes. One year, his work took him to New Zealand to meet with Arthur Lydiard, a fellow coach who, despite being self-educated, was helping to produce world-class athletes. While there, Bowerman accepted an invitation from Lydiard to join Auckland Joggers Club. Off he went on a trail run and to his surprise, Bowerman found it *tough*. Writing in *Jogging: A Physical Fitness Program for All Ages*, Bowerman's official guide on jogging published a few years after this trip, he said: 'I did quite well for the first half-mile. Then, just as I was beginning to feel a little winded and expect a slightly slower pace, the group turned up to cross a shoulder of the mountain without any slackening at all. By twos and threes the joggers passed me, helping me work from the middle to almost the tail end of the crowd. Then I noticed a nice gentleman graciously matching his pace to my own . . . By the time we had reached the mid-point of the trail, he led me on a short-cut down the mountain which brought us back to the finish at almost the same time as everyone else. It saved public embarrassment, but not private.'

After this Bowerman devised his own jogging plan, and it's said that after only a month of jogging Bowerman returned to the US lighter and being able to 'jog' for longer. He shared his results with the sports media and included an invite to fellow Oregon residents to 'come jogging' at the University of Oregon athletics track. This meeting created the city's own joggers' club and Bowerman was hooked. He even went so far as to enlist the help of a cardiologist, Waldo Harris, to investigate the benefits of jogging. Their findings led to Bowerman writing his aforementioned book, which mapped out how far, fast and how often to jog. It caught the attention of the media and the book went on to sell over a million copies. From then on, jogging was officially a *thing*.

Today, jogging has rightfully evolved into running and it's more popular than ever. According to Couch to 5K[10], published by Public Health England, more than 2 million people have completed their journey to successfully running 5,000 metres. And given my previous admission that I've quit halfway through a run more times than I can count, I've become fascinated with working out what it is that keeps so many people moving forward. For me, it was discovering that, although so many view running as a solitary sport, it doesn't have to be.

True, many people enjoy running alone. Often it's an invaluable portion of me-time and an opportunity to clear your head. But for others it's a necessary evil. And for those people, like me, it pays to hark back to what got Bowerman hooked on 'jogging' in the first place. It was the community. It was the support he got running through New Zealand when times got tough.

Now, running clubs are not new. There are plenty in London alone. However, to many the scene can seem hyper-competitive and unwelcoming. As a beginner, breaking into these clubs for the first time can be intimidating. Just as common, however, are clubs that have a way of making everything better, and you'll wonder why it took you so long to build up the courage to take the plunge in the first place.

For me that moment came on one drab Monday in 2018. An invitation to Track Life LDN forced my hand to sample running with a crew. On my way there, I started to regret my decision. Despite being fitter than your average Joe I still fretted about being the slowest on the track and was concerned that my lack of running lingo – at the time I didn't know my split times from my spikes – would be just like wearing a big white label with the words 'not a real runner' on it. Of course, these irrational thoughts were just more examples of my anxious state of mind and (you guessed it) they were a completely pointless use of mental energy.

That's not to say my arrival went smoothly. In fact, as I checked in with reception and flew through the turnstile to head towards the session, the string on my running coat got caught. I was trapped, and a tailback of eager runners began building up behind me as I gradually turned a deeper shade of purple through embarrassment. How was I meant to clear the hurdles on the track if I couldn't even navigate the entrance turnstile?

As the session got under way my anxiety eased and I became more myself with every step. I quickly realised that no one gave a crap about my agility or ability to A-skip because they were far too focused on their own running drills. Before long I had shrugged off the self-imposed 'newbie' title. Then came the main part of the session: a lung-busting running pyramid. If you, like me at the time, have no idea what the hell that entails, allow me to elaborate. A pyramid session involves starting with a rep at a certain time or distance; in my session it was distance. Then, each rep increases in distance (or time) until a maximum (i.e. the tip of the pyramid) is reached. You then do the opposite and decrease the distance of each rep until you reach the starting point again. I quickly did the maths for that session: 100m + 200m + 300m + 400m + 300m + 200m + 100m. Basically, we were about to do a mile's worth of sprints. I wasn't sure whether to laugh or cry.

Determined not to look like a dweeb for the second time that evening, I toed the starting line. Three, two, one . . . Go! To my delight, I kept pace. Together with the other members of the 'sexy' pace group ('there's no such thing as slow,' the coaches say) we managed to get through the first rep. With every stride, I dug deeper. I pumped my arms like Tom Cruise and practised the knee drive I'd learned from the earlier drills. I kept the focus on the finish line and gave everything I had to get there. And when I did, my work wasn't done – despite being desperate not to expel the contents of my stomach all over my new Nikes.

At this run club, when not doing your own work, you help others get theirs done. 'One thing all of our runners have in common is their passion for self-improvement,' Omar Mansour, co-founder of the club, told me afterwards. 'A lot of traditional running clubs can be elitist or cliquey. We promote a community feel within our club,' added Rory Knight, Track Life's other co-conspirator. What this means is the atmosphere is the best kind of happy-clappy. Run your best 200m? High-five for that. Came last but completed it? Another high-five. It was this initiation into run clubs that made me realise there really *is* a time and pace for everyone.

For the next year, I ran with the Track Life crew as much as I could. I enjoyed being in an environment where all abilities ran together. When there's always someone slower that needs your support and, equally, someone faster to put you in your place, there's no room for ego. I got fitter, I got faster and here's

the best bit: for two hours each week while running I relin-
quished power over to the coaches. I let go and did as I was
told. I was switched on, but I could also switch off. It was bliss.

Since then, I've run with other crews and I've always walked
away with mental and physical boons from running in a group.
In fact, I'm writing this chapter only hours after finishing my
local Parkrun. The run began with a celebration of the parkrun
devotees who'd hit a milestone (you get a t-shirt for reaching
10, 50, 100, 250 runs). The runners who congregated in Hillyfields
– a South London park – whooped and cheered for their cardio
crew. It's only when you join them that you realise, quite apart
from race times and weight-loss ambitions, this is what running
is all about. They also cheer first timers and tourists – less to
do with running achievement and more just being there at all.

TRACKING DOWN YOUR TRIBE

It's easy to come up with excuses to not try a club. They cost
money, you have to travel to get there, you might be the slowest
in the group. But these drawbacks will be forgotten when you're
rewarded with the benefits. According to Strava,[11] those who
exercise in groups last 10 per cent longer and cover 21 per cent
more distance than those who go it alone. Plus, UK Active[12]
say group workouts provide the highest Social Value (the value
to the communities that they serve) per person, at over £430
in recent years.

Around the globe, running clubs exist in many forms. You'll
notice that many have the term 'harrier' in their title, which is
a general nickname for cross-country runners. A bit of running
history for you: this term originates from a 19th-century
schoolboy game that evolved into a worldwide running club

that typically meets for a 6-mile run with alcohol before, during and after. If this sounds like your type of running tribe then skip straight to details on the Hash House Harriers on p.62 – if not, stick with me.

To find a crew that speaks to you, let me first suggest thinking about what you'd like to improve upon. There's little value in joining a track club if you're great at going fast but are forever finding excuses to cut your long run short. Instead, look for a club that progresses a weekly long run. This will help you build up your distance. Want to get faster over 5k? Choose a tribe that runs in pace groups and chase the faster group up ahead.

6 OF THE BEST UK RUNNING CLUBS

Whether you're in England, Scotland or Wales, it's easy to locate athletic friends using the 'club finder' function set up by the national sporting governing bodies.

scottishathletics.org.uk/athletes/get-involved/club-finder/
welshathletics.org/en/club
englandathletics.org/find-an-athletics-club/

Additionally, Run Together (runtogether.co.uk/about/) is a handy resource for runners of all abilities. Set up by England Athletics, it's a one-stop-shop listing running programmes, groups and routes, and offers the ability to filter by 'paid', 'free' and running opportunities for 'guided runners'.

And then there are the new breed of running clubs that offer immersive experiences. Let me introduce you to my edit of the clubs going the extra mile.

'Great things never came from comfort zones'

Run Dem Crew

Spend a night or two in any city and you'll no doubt watch an urban running club whizz by. Travelling as one body, they dodge pedestrians and buses. But no club you see will turn heads quite as fast as Run Dem Crew. They look *good*. Now a stalwart on the London running scene, this club was started 14 years ago by Charlie Dark, who says running 'literally saved my life'. Today, he's gathered hundreds of members who meet each week for city cardio while exchanging creative chat and ideas. If you like to think on your feet, this is for you.

rundemcrew.com

LDN Brunch Club

Will you run for brunch? Join this crew whose mission is to end at a different brunch spot each week while helping you get race ready. During marathon season there are run leaders and pacers on hand to help you progress your speed over longer distances.

ldnbrunchclub.co.uk

Lululemon Global Free Run Club

Globally, this is one of the largest free run clubs on Strava. You start and finish at one of the brand's many stores and at some stores there's focus on 'backpackers' – that's slow and steady runners who normally bring up the rear. It's the run club for when you're just finding your feet, wherever you may be.

lululemon.co.uk/community

Tracklife LDN

Sedentary office workers with hunched shoulders and in need of a blowout, this one is for you. Master the art of glute activation while honing in on your running posture and technique, then go really, really fast. Trainers Rory Knight and Omar Mansour will help rectify the wrongs of sitting down while teaching you how to finesse the form points that are key to running faster.

tracklifeldn.com

GoodGym

It's now possible to do good for others while being good to your body. Join one of the 54 GoodGym run clubs nationwide that offer an altruistic take on getting fit. Every week they run to help with local community projects, and run back, all within 90 minutes. One week you might make sandwiches for the homeless, the next you'll paint a fence at the community centre. It's charity meets cardio.

goodgym.org/group-runs

Hash House Harriers

They've been described as a 'drinking club with a running problem', as this crew always start at the pub. What happens next is a trail run with runners following directions marked in either flour or chalk on the ground. It's non-competitive and some runs have a mid-trail stop for more drinks. This happens around the world and is a good way to meet locals when travelling. Insider tip: new shoes are frowned upon and there is a special ceremony for anyone caught wearing them. There's nothing boring about this crew.

londonhash.org

SOCIAL SUPPORT

To realise your running potential with no location or time constraints, I suggest dipping a toe into the world of virtual running. A bit Matrix-y, yes, but well worth it. Just like IRL clubs, virtual running clubs offer both community and coaching. And they don't discriminate either: whether you're heading out for your first run or training for a race, there is a digital crew for you.

3 ways to get connected:

Strava

With more than 64 million members around the world, Strava offers miles and miles of inspiration at your fingertips. In 2018 alone, women uploaded more than 90 million runs to the platform and those who'd set themselves a run goal using the app were 15 per cent more likely to achieve it. Plus, it's super simple to set up. Simply download the app, create an account and start searching for friends to follow. By doing so, you'll populate your feed with recent runs of your virtual crew and you can give them kudos on their activity and leave comments.

Go one step further and you can also join a 'club'. Hosted by locals as well as brands like Garmin, these virtual crews bring like-minded people together, for example The Weekly 5K Club. Hosted by Ultra Runner Susie Chan. This digital crew all run (you guessed it) 5k each week, and post their efforts to the group. Drop in on the leaderboard to see who's topping the charts for the most weekly mileage or look at the recent posts to see photos, links and comments from other runners that can push you to go further.

Get inspired: to train like an athlete you can also visit strava. com/pros for a list of professionals using the sweatwork. Here, you can easily find and follow your cardio crush.

Insider tip: since time began humans have benefited mentally from the approval of others, and in the running community it's no different. So make friends with Strava's secret Mass Kudos feature. After a mass participation race or event click on the section to see the full list of runners who completed the same route (or race) as you. Now give your phone a quick shake and you'll give kudos to *everyone*. Share the love – it's a winning feature, even if you didn't win the race.

Nike Run Club app

If you lack the motivation to lace up, let Nike help. Since its launch, Nike Run Club has inspired thousands of runners to *just do it*. How? By building a free app that offers in-run cheers from friends and ways to personalise and post your running photos. Add stickers and your stats, then share your success with your running fam.

Get inspired: use the guided runs to ensure you're never lonely or lack direction on a run again. You can choose between virtual coaching for running firsts – think, your first long run or first speed session – or choose to run with Headspace and use cardio to clear your mind.

Insider tip: you'll know from chapter 1 why running your trainers into the ground might be good for your bank account but isn't advisable for your feet, so use the app to track how many miles you've run in every pair of running shoes you own – even the ones that aren't Nike.

Runkeeper

There are more than 45 million people on Runkeeper – that's more than the population of Canada. It's quite the crew. Since launching 11 years ago this running network has tirelessly updated their offering, which is liked by runners around the world. At the time of writing, more than half a million photos are using #runkeeper on Instagram, which is handy for an unending source of inspo.

Get inspired: to help you go the distance, sign up to a virtual race and don't forget to celebrate your progress with friends.

Insider tip: choose Goal Coach for guidance in setting running goals that are right for you. It's as close as you'll get to a personal running coach without having to reach for your credit card.

ADD TO THE SWEATWORK

If you love running but aren't into sweaty selfies, you're not alone. The running community is creative when it comes to celebrating their sweat. To join the conversation, try these three types of posts on Instagram and Twitter:

Medal Monday
The name is a big giveaway: you post your recently awarded race medal the Monday after it happened.

Flat lays
Pre-race flat lay photos are a popular running ritual. Unlike brunch flat lays which often require climbing onto a café chair for that perfect angle, annoying your friends in the process, the running flat lay is easy to achieve. Simply lay out your bib, shoes, socks, watch, gels – essentially anything you'll use on race day. For the best shot, lay in natural light and on carpet it doesn't reflect.

Run routes

As you've read, many running apps offer the ability to brand up your run route and share it to IG. It's a great resource for sharing your journey with local runners. Alternatively, you could get creative like 'Dick Run Clare', who is using Instagram to share her penis-shaped running routes. Each to their own.

Top running hashtags to follow

Throughout my running journey I've often called on social media for motivation and inspiration, and hashtags are the lazy (but incredibly useful) way to find it, from discovering runners who endured frozen beards and hair in pursuit of their winter miles, to the women giving taboos the bump and running while pregnant. This is how I search social media to fuel my own success.

#wellfar
#runningcommunity
#medalmonday
#sundayrunday
#longrun
#instarunners
#seenonmyrun
#Londonrunners
#womensrunningcommunity
#halfmarathontraining
#marathontraining
#runningislife
#thesweatlife
#tracklife
#runningismytherapy
#runhappy

Tip: When you sign up for a race, start following the event hashtag. This is an easy way to connect with others taking on the distance. Like, comment and engage and you'll find that others will do the same. In no time you'll have built yourself a virtual support crew.

Your Chapter 2 Action Plan

- Use the national athletics databases to find a running club close to home

- Pick a club that will suit your goals. Track for speed. Harrier for fun

- Get app happy and join an online community like Strava

- Post your kit flat lays and comment on people's posts to share love and support

- Follow the race hashtag as soon as you sign up, to easily link up with runners IRL

CHAPTER 3

Now You're Up And Running

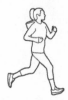

My Journey

In ancient Greece, women were forbidden to compete in the Olympic Games. Today, female running accomplishments are front and centre creating headlines around the world. Which is made even more remarkable when you realise that we don't have genetics on our side.

If you were asked to 'run like a girl' what would you do? Slow down? Flap your arms and play up to the gender stereotype? I remember tweenage boys shouting 'you run like a girl'. They'd shout these four words at their slower friend desperately trying not to sink into the boggy cross-country course. It didn't matter that he was putting in as much effort as he could muster, he was slow and ungainly and that meant he ran like a girl. Simple as that.

For years, the phrase 'like a girl' has fed into the notion that, when it comes to being physically active, women and men are not the same. In most cases men are bigger and stronger and, especially over short distances, find it easier to go faster. It's bloody infuriating and something I've felt first hand. A few years ago I spent two months getting myself ready to take on the Great South Run. My training cycle was near perfect and I walked towards the startline in Portsmouth with a confident spring in my step. However, my husband (boyfriend at the time) did not train. He did one 'long run' to check that it was humanly possible for him to run longer than 5k and, as he survived it, he headed straight into his taper. This consisted only of 10m intervals from the couch to the kitchen for biscuits because #carbloading.

And so, race day came and off we went. As we ran along the seafront through the historic dockyard we were shoulder-to-shoulder, pacing pretty evenly without even trying. When the winds blew *and they did* because it was a really blustery day on the coast, we'd grimace at each other while sharing a knowing look of 'this is bloody hard'. I hadn't run a race with anyone else before, at least not side-by-side with someone I started with, so I enjoyed the company.

Then, around 8 miles, with only two left to go, Ted took out his headphones and shouted: 'I really need to finish so I'm going to run on.' At the time, this didn't faze me because a wild idea had popped into my head: he was digging really, effing deep as he wanted to get to the finish line early and get down on one knee. *He was going to propose!* For the next 18 minutes, as the winds made it hard to keep course and my energy levels continued to tank, I visualised him saying the magic four words: will you marry me? It gave me renewed energy and mental grit that I hadn't felt all race. As I ran down the final straight I kept thinking, He'll come into focus soon, but with 50, 40, 20, 10 metres to go there was no sign. I was confused. Then I told myself that of course he wouldn't be on the actual finish line because that wouldn't be allowed – he'll be just after the medals. Silly me. But as I got to the end of the trestle tables there was no Ted. I scanned the crowd for a good 15 minutes before I eventually tracked him down. He was on his way to the pub. There was no proposal. Instead, Ted had simply become exhausted by the monotonous action of putting one foot in front of the other and sped up to get the race over and done with. When he told me this I wasn't sure what I was most disappointed about: the lack of diamonds or the fact that I'd given everything I possibly could during that race, yet it still wasn't enough to beat my boyfriend who had done one solitary training run. As you can imagine, I ordered a very large red wine.

To understand how my husband – who I love dearly but who is more used to running out of money than he is actually running – managed to run negative splits in a race that he hadn't trained for, it's time to recruit science. The simple fact is, Ted had biology on his side.

Heart size

A man's heart is 20–25 per cent larger than the average woman's, giving them an advantage. Their bigger left ventricle is better able to pump oxygenated blood around the body to be used in their muscles. During a race this helps men to run faster for longer.

Body fat

We know that you can be both fat and fit; however, when it comes to running, fat can slow you down. While it's of no concern to your recreational athlete, it's a consideration for pros looking to run like Radcliffe. Women are predisposed to hold an additional 5–10 per cent body fat compared to men. We need this extra layer for child-bearing. Several studies[13] have examined the relationship between increased weight and running performance and the outcome is this: predictably, excess weight results in a worse performance. So, on runs shorter than a marathon, men have the advantage but when it comes to ultras, this biological win actually starts to work against them, and women can push on from strength to strength.

Hormones

The chemical messengers (hormones) in men and women vary, obviously. In the male body the primary hormone is testosterone, famous for stimulating muscle mass development. It also plays a part in the concentration of red blood cells, and haemoglobin, which are critical for transporting oxygen around the body. In the female body the primary hormone is oestrogen. Among its many functions is that it stimulates fat accumulation. It's thought that this difference in hormones means that on average male blood can carry around 11 per cent more oxygen than female blood. This helps to make men more efficient runners.

Injuries

We women are at a significantly higher risk of injury than men. Specifically, we're more prone to knee and shin injuries. The reasons include running gait, a wider pelvis, menstrual cycles and training habits. Thankfully, an awareness of bone health, regular core-strengthening exercises, a well-structured training plan and being aware of your miles and menstrual cycle can help to mitigate this biological drawback.

But far from a shortlist of excuses, these are motivators and scientific proof of women's incredible ability to outrun the odds. Biology may be stacked against us in many ways, but since 2001 female marathon runners have only become faster, shaving an average of four minutes from their race time. To run like a girl is to make positive steps even when we've not been dealt a winning hand; it's to run with guts and it's something to be proud of. With the right tools and knowledge women can make real strides. Which is where our next expert comes in.

'If you see me collapse, pause my Garmin'

Follow The Leader

Anthony 'Fletch' Fletcher is a personal trainer specialising in biomechanics. He is the founder of Onetrack run club and works with elite runners and everyday athletes alike, coaching regular gym-goers and Olympic hopefuls. Whatever goal you're chasing, he can help you get there – and he is here to tell you how.

STAYING TRUE TO FORM

The first thing you need to accept is that everyone runs differently. If you implement concrete running rules then you can lose time and effort obsessing over details that are nearly impossible to correct. For example, your arm might come across the body simply because that's the way you're put together. Trying to 'fix' and adjust that can create more problems than it solves, especially if you're new to running and the brain is already having to get used to a lot of newly-moving parts.

Instead of hard-and-fast rules, it's better and easier to keep some general ideas in mind.

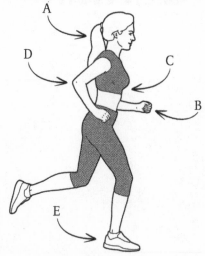

Firstly, *relax*. Without thinking, the effort of running can cause the muscles in the neck to fire up with every step, as they attempt to stabilise your shoulders. That tension ends up being exhausting, expending unnecessary effort. Mentally check in from time to time to see where your shoulders are – if they're up under your ears, you're too tense. Let them drop (A). Do the same with your jaw, forehead, wrists and fingers. To keep your hands loose, imagine you're running cradling an egg in either hand (B). All tensing really does is to show other people that you're working hard. In treadmill classes you see people grimacing as they go all-out, but that makes no difference to performance. It's a waste of effort.

Next, consider that running can take a toll on your lower back. One thing that can help there is to run with a slight brace in your core to create some protective tension. I'm talking about a 2/10 effort, tensing slightly in the back of your mind (C). That will then become second nature.

Use your elbows more than you think. Actually push your elbow back slightly as that same knee goes forward (D). Especially for heavier runners and beginners, you need to combat a lot of upper-body rotation because you haven't yet got the coordination between the upper and lower body. If you don't push back, the elbow sticks into the ribs and you end up twisting your upper body to drive your legs, which will exhaust your core. Pumping your arms will help to offset this.

Finally, lots of runners, especially when they're fatigued, struggle with the runner shuffle, where you barely pick your feet up off the ground. If you can feel that's the case, focus on lifting your knees a little higher (E) so you have slightly more time in the air for your foot to get in the right position.

DON'T GO ON STRIKE

A few years ago, the emergence of barefoot running – you know, the shoes with incredibly thin soles – started a whole new conversation. It introduced a lot of people to the difference between forefoot striking and heel striking. Barefoot running, and consequently switching to a forefoot strike, got a lot of press, promising to help you go faster by running 'naturally'. The problem is, there's nothing natural about manipulating the way your foot strikes the ground. It's another example of giving yourself too many things to think about with barely any scientific justification.

And though my advice when it comes to foot strike boils down to 'ignore it and run', knowledge is important and an explainer may help to stop you getting confused by marketing spiel and click-bait articles on the internet.

Heel strike

The heel strike is exactly as you would imagine. It means striking the floor with your heel with every stride. You do it when you walk all the time. And there's a natural mechanism we do from the heel strike called pronation, which is the natural shock absorption of the foot (remember chapter 1?), helping us to keep moving forward. Simply put, heel striking is what we use for the slowest of speeds, and we roll from the back of the foot to the front of the foot.

Midfoot strike

The midfoot strike is landing in the midfoot, slightly further forward. It's not landing totally flat footed, but with a slight heel raise and that's more of a transitional strike, and is common in someone who is running at a semi-race pace. You can also switch to midfoot strike subconsciously when you're protecting yourself from something, like a soreness or a change in terrain.

Forefoot strike

The forefoot strike, then, is about speed. It provides maximum shock absorption and maximum elasticity through the body to get you moving forward faster.

Swapping between footstrikes, therefore, is not something you need to concern yourself with. Instead, it's a natural thing that your body is dialled in to adapt, depending on effort. The brain is the most advanced computer in the world, but there are two sides to it. One is the genius in the background that doesn't say anything while quietly getting on with things. Then you've got the other one, the podium guy, the conscious brain who is constantly saying, 'We should do this!' All the while, the guy in the background is shouting, 'Stop interfering!' We're obsessed with trying to overrule the subconscious, but the vast majority of the time it's better to let your body get on with it.

THE NEED FOR SPEED?

A simple definition of cadence – a word you may hear a lot in certain training plans or advice articles – is how many steps you're taking per minute. It's the same as the BPM of a song.

The common mistake with cadence comes with speed, and when you're running slowly (beginners take note!). You feel like you don't need to take as many strides per minute. As your cadence drops you end up bounding from one foot to the other and this results in a lot of contact time between foot and floor.

The longer the contact time, the more time you're spending on each leg and the faster you'll wear out.

It sounds counter-intuitive, but by increasing your cadence and taking more steps you actually reduce contact time and can take the pressure off your body. Imagine I'm passing you a hot cup of tea and you have to hold it for 10 seconds once. Imagine then holding it for 2 seconds, five times. Then see how many times you can repeat each process with the piping hot cuppa before it becomes painful. You'll find that the increased cadence reduces the burn.

Most of the research into cadence and running performance has been done on elite runners. So, when people say you need to be hitting 180 steps per minute for optimum performance, well, it doesn't work like that. Elite runners are often 5'7" and weigh 55 kilos. They're not your average runner and so prescribing yourself their protocols is no guarantee of success.

What's better is to gradually manipulate cadence a little bit to work out what feels more comfortable to you. The less pressure you feel, and the less load through the joints, can help with injury prevention. There's even science suggesting that an increase in cadence of 15 per cent can lead to a reduction in load through the knees by 35 per cent, and that's huge because knees are the number-one complaint for runners.

> **The average recreational runner has a cadence anywhere between 150 and 170 spm.**

DIFFERENT TYPES OF RUN

If you download a plan from the internet or rip one out of a magazine, then you're likely to see your training runs broken down into certain categories throughout the week. This is your decoder.

Long run

This is an exercise in spending more time on your feet and, especially if you're a beginner, then your pace should be irrelevant. You should aim to cover a set distance.

Extra time on feet allows your body the time it needs to develop and for those little stabiliser muscles in your joints to adapt to the strain. And so long runs for beginners don't actually need to be that long, they just need to be steady.

And that's a problem sometimes, especially for beginners going into a marathon plan. You might think that you need to get up to running 10k or further right away. But that's not true. You need to get it into your head that the 2k run exists and it's worthwhile because that's still 2,000 steps that you need to take. Long doesn't have to be long, it can just mean the longest run you've done so far. And then you build it up over time, which is what your body needs – time. A trick I use with running newbies is to swap the emphasis from distance to time. Say you're going to go out for half an hour, and that's it, no matter how far you travel in that time.

Tempo run

As the first one is about spending time on your feet, this one is about spending time at your race pace. If you're working towards a certain time for an upcoming run or race then you'll know that you need to hit a certain minutes-per-mile speed to get across the line in time – for example, a 9:30 minutes per mile to run a 5k in under 30 minutes. As you progress to different races, you'll have different paces for 5k, 10k, half marathon or marathon. There's also nothing to stop you swapping between measuring your pace in minutes per mile or minutes per kilometre; it's what works for you.

However, at the beginning of your plan you may only be able to hold that pace for 1K. Your tempo run is an opportunity to spend more and more time going more quickly. Because you can only hold these new paces for a short time initially, you can start introducing 'fartlek' to your tempo runs. Loosely translated from Swedish, this means 'speed play' and encourages you to fill a session with easy, medium and fast paces. Over the course of your 40-minute training run you can gradually increase your time at race pace before dropping back, recovering and then going again.

These tempo run intervals don't have to be done individually, either. You can play around with it during your long runs, too. You could do your first 5k of 20k super easy, then the next 5k at your race pace and finish with a slow 10k, spending time on your feet. It can make long runs more interesting, which is important. When long runs are boring it can increase the risk of injury because you start to get absent minded, your cadence decreases and you settle into a weird rhythm. The change of speeds can keep the focus in place.

When you then get closer to your race date you can look to go faster and start hitting 105, 110, 115 per cent of your race pace. That's because you're going to start bringing the volume down as you start to taper, so you need to put the intensity up to get the training effect that'll lead to fitness gains.

Sprint sessions

These are a good way of breaking up longer runs to make them less time-consuming, but also to go beyond race pace more often and help you to find it easier going fast. So, if you're training for a 5k then try this, resting between the 400m stints:

- 1k warm up
- race pace for 400m x 10

These sprints are an effective way to tap into the higher heart rates that you're not getting from your long runs. By hitting 80–90 per cent of your maximum heart rate (that's near max effort) you'll enter what's called the anaerobic zone. This zone improves your 'anaerobic capacity', increasing your lactate threshold. That means the intensity you can run at before a build up of lactic acid puts on the brakes. You can't train here for long, which is why it's best to break them down into sprints, but the cardio benefits will mean that you can go faster for longer on your next tempo and long run. The gritted teeth will be worth it.

Recovery sessions

To get a little fitness in the bank without overloading yourself, add a recovery session into your week. You can even take the load off the body and do it on a bike. For that, go at a rate of perceived exertion (RPE) of 4/10 and hold that for 30 minutes.

> TIP: As you start out, it's important to change what you do every week. You might do a little bit more on one week, then less the next week. Then build up for two weeks and then back off again. The key is to keep it varied so you don't fall into a rhythm too early and get bored.

Heart Rate Zones

There are three main training zones that can help you to target different goals. They are a percentage of your max heart rate, which you calculate by working out 220 minus your age. If you want to follow along on your Fitbit or other tracker, these are the breakdowns:

60–70 per cent: the fat-burning zone. Easy training at a conversational pace. Good for long runs and spending more time on your feet. This commonly matches the 'easy' term in running training plans and would measure a 4–6 as a rate of perceived exertion (that's how hard you find it out of 10, basically).

70–80 per cent: the aerobic zone. The most effective zone for improving cardiovascular fitness and building stamina. This is the zone you'll spend most time in during steady runs and resistance workouts.

80–90 per cent: the anaerobic zone. As explained, you'll be working at a fast pace and breathing hard. This zone improves your anaerobic capacity to increase the amount of time you can spend running at race pace.

PICKING A RACE PACE

As you graduate up from 5k to take on greater distances, often the temptation is to go faster as well as further. It's the reason that in a lot of running plans you see this term 'race pace'. Essentially, that is the average speed you need to run at between start and finish line, and it's often pitched in minutes per mile. For example, if you're really going for it and hope to hit a 1h45m half marathon, then you need to run every mile of the 13.1 distance at an 8-minute pace.

But let me slow you down. Taking an interest in race pace, whether it's plastered over your running plan or not, really depends on what your goal is. If you want to simply complete a distance then running at a race pace shouldn't be a part of the training. It should just be time on feet and learning to run for the enjoyment that's in it. If it's your first race, then what's far more important than trialling race pace in training is to first make sure you do every long run and make running a habit. Adding in race paces (especially if you come up short) is just another opportunity to give up.

The only time you ever use a race pace is when you are really set on a time. As mentioned, it can then serve as a guide to the type of speeds you need to achieve (and get used to) in your tempo runs.

Race Pace Calculator:
Sub-30min 5k: 9:40 per mile
Sub-45min 10k: 7:15 per mile
Sub-2hr half marathon: 9:09 per mile
Sub-4hr marathon: 9:00 per mile

While 'race pace' can be useful in training, sticking to it religiously on race day can cause complications. Think about starting your first marathon in Pen 5, for example. You're not going to get up to race pace for the first couple of miles because you need to work your way through the crowds. It's a totally different experience to testing out what an 8-minute mile feels like at a quiet Parkrun.

Then again, whether you should even get up to race pace early in a race is up for debate. As coaches we see a consistent drop-off in people who start too quickly. If you get rushed along by an attack of Big Race Energy early on, the drop-off rate after halfway is severe. I always advise my runners to start more slowly. The golden number is to fiddle around with your race pace and account for running about 15 seconds slower than that pace for the first half. Then that will leave you enough in the tank to step up to or beyond that speed for the second half.

The learning really is that there is no magic number that will get you a PB. Picking a race pace is a guide, not a guarantee.

TAKE A DEEP BREATH NOW

No matter how fast you decide to go, or how many steps you take per minute, there is another, far more basic potential stumbling block. Breathing. When it comes to breathing, there are two simple mistakes you can make. Thankfully, they're equally simple to overcome. Here are the ins and outs:

1. Thinking that it's something you can control

Breathing is a mechanism of the unconscious and therefore is a job that you have very little control over. There are lots of mechanisms that we are not aware of when we're running, but because breathing is on the surface it's brought to the attention of your conscious brain. You can try to control your breathing – be that nasal breathing only, or two seconds in, two seconds out – but these will make no difference to performance, rather they're just a way of giving yourself something to focus on, so that you feel in control. You'd be just as well served by ignoring the way you're breathing, focusing on something else and letting the body do its job. It has taken millions of years to create that breathing mechanism as you run; it's unlikely you'll be able to improve upon that now!

2. Panicking when getting out of breath

Getting out of breath is nothing to fear. It's a symptom of hard work. However, especially for beginners, the shortness of breath and panting can feel like the symptoms of a panic attack. Breathing rate increases to compensate and fuel all the muscle activity that's happening when you run. Hydrogen is produced in the muscles and the respiratory system is trying to get rid of it. It's a natural thing, and it will get easier as you train and become a fitter, more efficient runner. In the moment, the best tactic is to take a big, deep breath and slow down. This will not only reduce the amount of hydrogen your body needs to process but also calm down your body and nervous system, which may help to get your breathing under control.

And finally, what about the dreaded stitch?

Incredibly, no one is really sure what a stitch is. Researchers Morton and Callister did a literary review of 15 years of science into Exercise-related Transient Abdominal Pain (jargon for a stitch)[14] and found that there was little evidence as to exactly what's happening. The suggestion is that it's an irritation of the abdominal and pelvic lining, the prevention of which starts in the gym. It's thought that strengthening your core muscles and training them to control dynamic movement can help to reduce irritation and therefore symptoms. Though the classic advice of not ploughing through large quantities of food and drink before heading out for a run also rings true. So save that meal as a post-run reward.

Your Chapter 3 Action Plan

- Don't obsess about form – running like a girl is a good thing. Just relaaaaaax

- Try upping your cadence slightly; you may find it takes some pressure off your joints

- Focus on time – not distance – for long runs, to get your body used to everything at the start

- Don't pick a race pace until you're ready, and then only use it as a training guide

- Include core exercises, such as planking, in your gym workouts to help prevent stitches when you run

CHAPTER 4

Food For Thought

My Journey

The relationship between food and body image is complicated. In comparison, the relationship between food and fitness is refreshingly simple. Having finally wrapped my head around this, I'm faster, healthier and a hell of a lot happier than I've ever been before.

I can still taste the first time that food became a source of torment, not nourishment. I was three years old and my sister had had enough of my constant bullying. She bit back and chased me around the house until she caught me and force-fed me a segment of orange. I desperately tried to spit it out while gagging on the awful, pithy, stringy stuff.

When this citrusy waterboarding was over I didn't just cry, I screamed the house down. To some, especially my sister, it was an overreaction, but three-year-old me didn't see it like that. Back then I didn't just dislike fruit, I was terrified of it.

The wet and juicy textures and sickly smells made my skin crawl, and just touching it would send me into a meltdown. 'As a baby I once made you eat mashed banana,' my mum later told me. 'But it was the first and last time – shortly after I'd shoved in the last mouthful you violently sicked up the lot.'

A few years after Orangegate there was another incident. I was at my childminder's, happily combing the hair of my Troll Doll when one of the other kids decided it would be funny to smarm tomato pips from his plate onto my arm. Well, more fool him. For the next two hours I howled and howled because a tomato had touched me. I can't remember what made me finally stop crying – exhaustion, perhaps – but I know we were never served cherry tomatoes for lunch again.

My dramatic reaction towards fruit and most vegetables, or 'disgust reflex' as experts call it, lasted well into my teens. I can recall plenty of mealtimes spent trying to peel boiled new potatoes at the dinner table because my mother refused to comply with my no-skin-on-food rule. My sister thought I was a brat while my mum, exhausted as most single parents are, just let it pass. Either way, my fear of, and consequent refusal to eat, vegetables made mealtimes a testing experience for everyone around me.

It wasn't until I was nearly 16 that I finally stopped freaking out about skins, pips and stringy bits. Actually, that's not strictly true as there are still foods today that I won't touch, like cucumber or melon; just the smell of them makes me retch. But thankfully for my husband and fellow diners, I no longer turn hysterical should I mistake cucumber for courgette, and I'll happily unwrap Parma ham from a melon before shoving it in my mouth. But back as a teen, my diet of meat and potatoes became meat, potatoes and green beans. From there I got really adventurous – I even branched out to a vegetable stir-fry – once the bean sprouts, water chestnuts and bamboo shoots had been removed, obviously. It was slow progress, but progress nonetheless.

Then at 20, after a bad breakup, that progress faltered. I moved cities, went into reverse and my disordered eating came back with a vengeance. My body confidence began to crumble: it started small, like a few Rice Krispies falling from the side of a crackle cake, but after one term at a new college, those small crumbs turned into big chunks and I fell apart.

For the first time in my life I fell victim to the negative self-talk that I now know affects so many people. This critical commentary about how I looked followed me everywhere. I spent every waking moment hyper-aware of my appearance and what I could do to edit it.

Before then, I'd barely contemplated that what you put into your body affects the way it looks and how it operates. I was late to puberty which meant I'd stayed quite small and slight through my teens. As such, I never had to deal with the awkward emergence of bouncy boobs replacing my childish chest. I ate chocolate-covered everything and it never showed. I could binge on whatever I liked and still fit into my Kappa popper tracksuit and spaghetti string vest.

So, at 20, when I decided to attempt to eat better to look better (I finally learned that five slices of half-and-half bread slathered with jam didn't constitute a balanced diet) I didn't realise I was running headfirst into my next episode of food chaos.

Paradoxically, my problems all started with a commitment to what I thought was healthy eating. I looked for lower-calorie foods and menu options that were light in fat. I ordered my burgers bunless and on nights out I would drink a Skinny Bitch (that's vodka, soda and lime). This progressed to buying books including *The South Beach Diet* that promoted cutting out carbs to elicit rapid weight loss. It also promised increased heart health, but let's be honest, that wasn't top of my agenda.

Numbers 1 through 10 on my agenda at that time was getting lean AF. I devoured the headlines that vilified carbs and really did believe that breaking up with bread was the shortcut to slim. The problem was, once I began scrutinising my food and its nutritional makeup, I couldn't stop. Rather than seeing the benefits of ingredients, I'd obsess over the sugar and fat content. It wasn't long before my carb-free diet became my dairy-free, low-fat, low-sugar diet, too. The scariest thing is that no one around me batted an eyelid. Eating clean was cool.

While some people could deploy these diets in a more measured way, I couldn't. My 'healthy eating' became extreme, and for the next 10 years I would suffer through a psychological eating disorder. Writing those words still makes me wince, shudder and look away in denial. Jordan Younger, AKA The Balanced Blonde once said: 'No one plans to develop an eating disorder,' and she's right. But life doesn't always go to plan.

According to Beat Eating Disorders,[15] more than 1.25 million people in the UK have an eating disorder. Of those, 75 per cent are female. However, the early warning signs of this illness often go unnoticed. For years, I ignored the signs. Despite knowing that eating multiple bowls of granola and then purging them all back up again wasn't normal, it became my normal. I'd regularly go to the gym fasted, and work out until I could burpee no more. Back at home I'd then binge on packets of cookies and family-size chocolate bars. Once full, I'd head to the toilet and throw it all back up again. I was one of the many adults who was simply unable to process the signs of an eating disorder; shockingly the average delay is three and a half years between falling ill and recognising that you have a problem.

Spotting an eating disorder early on is rare. Out of 2,000 adults surveyed by Beat, nearly 80 per cent were not able to name a psychological symptom. And yet, physical signs of eating disorders are often the last symptoms to show, happening once the mental illness is ingrained. It's why many of you, I'm sure, can't understand why I couldn't see that being sick after bingeing on food was problematic. Well, that's because by then it was already too late. I'd been wrestling with these issues in my mind for years and lost. By the time I looked up from having my head in the toilet bowl, I couldn't help it.

To be honest, the only reason I finally faced up to my issues and confided in a close family member was because I got caught out. We were on holiday in Ibiza and I'd been spotted going to the toilet for a third time during dinner. I had a choice: I either admit the truth or lie and have my family believe that I had a Class A drug problem. I chose to break my silence on my bulimia.

Understanding eating disorders if you've never suffered from one can be baffling. Comprehending why anyone would go that far isn't easy. The only way I know to explain it is that, yes, I knew it was bad, but what was bigger than the fear I felt for the damage I was doing to my body was the disgust I felt looking at myself in the mirror. I no longer saw my true self. Instead, all I saw was my body in visceral detail, and my mind was whirring, one step ahead and already plotting how it was going to shave off inches from my thighs and arms, and telling me what I could and couldn't eat for the next 48 hours. It did this because at some point my brain had linked food and self-worth. And it's the same for millions of other people.

This is made even more distressing when you consider the UK's troubled relationship with body confidence. Only 6 per cent of the women surveyed by *Women's Health*[16] said they had high body confidence, while the Dove Choose Beautiful survey[17] found that only 4 per cent of women feel beautiful. It's this fragility that makes us so susceptible to destructive relationships with food. The distaste for the skin that we're in is contributing to a rise in eating disorders. Shockingly, in the past decade the number of patients admitted to hospital suffering from these illnesses has doubled.

After my admission in Ibiza, I thought life would get better. I thought that by saying the words I would magically become fixed. I believed I would be too ashamed to puke up my food again and I would finally recognise the severity of the situation. I wasn't and I didn't. Even when later that year I confided in two friends, thinking the extra eyes on me would help me to break my binge-purge eating patterns, nothing changed. For months I continued on with this behaviour, spending unnecessary money on food. I squandered my weekly budget on snacks and then watched as they – along with my self-worth – were flushed down the drain. There were times when I managed to break the cycle and I'd go weeks or months without doing myself harm, and I thought I was 'recovered', but then when I experienced change, stress or disappointment the disorder worked itself back into my life.

Throughout all of this, there were more problems lurking in the background. When I wasn't gorging on granola or processed snacks I masked my disordered eating tendencies by subscribing to the latest new-age food cult to hit the internet. I'd tell everyone this new way of eating was the route to better health, increased energy and glowing skin – not that I really gave a shit about that part; I was on a mission to get thin. Because, when I looked in the mirror I didn't see the abs that so many people often reference – a genetic perk that I get from my mum (thanks, Mum!) – but the small pockets of fat that squished between my bra strap and armpit. I didn't see the strong legs that had carried me over a half marathon finish line, but the lack of a thigh gap and cellulite on my bum. I was deluded by what a healthy body should look like and so snacked on quick-fix advice to iron out my self-perceived flaws.

That's why in 2016 I found myself with a mouth that stank like nail polisher remover, headaches so painful I had to call in sick to work and constipation so chronic that I was concerned that my faeces would eventually force their way out of the opposite end. I'm talking about the time that I went keto. It was hellish. For two weeks I stuck to the extremely low-carb food plan in order to force my body to burn fat, not carbohydrates. As I weighed everything I ate to ensure I consumed no more than 20g of carbs a day, I would remember my PT at the time and his roster of clients. His Instagram was full of bikini models who were so lean that a strong wind would blow them over. They looked super-human, like flesh-coloured Avatars – there wasn't an ounce of excess flesh. And if the Skinny Bitch Collective could do it, then why couldn't I?

Well, apart from the side effects I've already referred to, not to mention urine that you could smell 2 metres away from the toilet, it only increased my avoidance of more food groups. Plus, there's a major flaw in this food plan: you can't pause keto. If, like me, you eat this way for two weeks and then give up because the temptation of pizza is too strong, when you next step on the scales a few days later you'll most likely register the same weight as you did before going keto. Naturally, this ended in a heavy dose of self-criticism and trash talk, which, inevitably, propelled me into the arms of yet another self-prescribed weight-loss plan.

What I wish I'd known before going keto is that the initial weight loss seen on the scales by going low-carb is not fat melting away, but the body ridding itself of excess water. So when you reverse your diet, your body restocks its empty reserves, and this once again shows up on the scales. Simply put, I never did lose fat, just water.

Not long after the keto catastrophe, I tried the raw vegan diet. While some people eat like this for ethical or environmental reasons, I of course ate nothing but raw vegetables to get lean. I chased the notion that if I got back down to 53kg (the lightest I've been as an adult) everything would be golden. So I set about filling my fridge and cupboards with nothing but vegetables, legumes, nuts, seeds and cold-pressed oils. For the first 48 hours I really enjoyed eating raw. I spiralised courgettes and made cashew pesto. I blended cauliflower and made a raw pizza. I even made raw carrot cake ice cream.

It was working until a few days of juicing, blending, soaking, sprouting and dehydrating blew up in my face, literally. I had such bad gas and bloating that the only way to relieve the pressure was to go to the disabled toilet at work and get myself into a downward dog. I spent 20 minutes burping and farting while at the same time contemplating how many toilet germs I was inhaling by having my nose so close to the bathroom floor. After that day, I threw out the spiraliser and Jason Vale's juice book and instead vowed to leave raw veganism to Miranda Kerr and co.

It would be a few more years until I truly understood the benefits of a balanced diet. I was still indoctrinated in the school of 'carbs make you fat' and was suffering as a result. On reflection, the fact that I once weighed broccoli to log its carb content on My Fitness Pal was a sign that all was not well. All the while I was still exercising hard and wondering why I had such sore muscles, felt fatigued and was SO. DAMN. HUNGRY.

And then, after a night out, this intense need for food came back to bite me.

I'd been out with friends in London and stumbled in some time after midnight. I just about managed to smear some face cleanser over my skin before passing out in my room. I'm not quite sure what happened between that moment and coming around in the kitchen, but all I know today is that, somehow, I'd managed to sleep walk to the fridge. Totally naked. The reason I know this is because, upon hearing weird scrabbling sounds in the kitchen, my best friend's boyfriend (my landlord) clambered out of bed to check it out. He was confronted with me, stark no-bollock naked hacking away at an unripe avocado. I'd obviously decided in my drunk, hungry sleep that I needed food and beelined for the fridge. To this day, we've laughed about it but I'm always quick to move the conversation on because, number one: who wants to revisit the story of their best mate's boyfriend seeing their fanny? And number two: the fact that drunken me chose an avocado as a snack is so cringingly wellness.

Thankfully, not long after The Night of the Avocado Fanny a new breed of nutrition advice landed. For once, the new recipe books and diet manuals weren't campaigning for more kale and turmeric, but instead championed the merits of carbohydrates for weight loss. Bob Harper (celebrity trainer and the guy from *America's Biggest Loser*) published *The Super Carb Diet*. In it, he explains how going from a Paleo diet to a carb-rich meal plan can help prevent constant food cravings and feelings of deprivation. This was also around the same time that Joe Wicks started to bust the myth that eating carbs after 6pm will make you fat. Further research by Stanford Prevention Research Center[18] in California agreed with Harper and Wicks: a low-carb diet is no better for life-long weight loss than a low-fat diet. The key is quality food.

Inspired, and intrigued by the new nutrition ideology, I chewed over the science. It turns out that after intense exercise the body's biggest concern is replacing energy stores (glycogen). Sure, it needs protein to repair muscles but if you don't restock your muscles with its favoured form of energy, then chances are your next workout will feel harder. Ideally you'd eat a 3:1 ratio of carbohydrates to protein after a workout. I hadn't been doing this. I'd removed oats, bananas and other forms of carbs from my post-workout shakes and instead chugged only protein powder and water. Without knowing it, I'd actually cut the food group that my body so desperately needed for intense exercise, and my AppleWatch recorded the results: my split times got slower, not faster. I'd unwittingly given myself a nutritional handicap.

Clearing up my confusion on carbs was a 'holy shit' moment. For years, I'd been led to believe they were bad. However, by understanding their function in a balanced diet I was able to stop seeing them as foe but a friend to my running. And when I started marathon training I truly understood their importance in fuelling success.

I'm not crediting running with curing my disordered eating habits – though I can happily report that my relationship with food has been far happier for around three years now – but from a situation where I was battling through the confusion of conflating food and body image, arming myself with the real nutritional knowledge that comes with fuelling fitness has helped no-end. Today, I don't put a label on my diet or subscribe to a plan. I eat mindfully, thinking about what fuel my body needs to carry out the tasks I ask of it. I believe there's a time and place for all foods, you just need to know why.

'Pain is just the French word for bread'

Follow The Leader

After working for the NHS, Anita Bean set up her own nutrition consultancy in 1990, specialising in sport and exercise nutrition and food writing. She has worked with the British Olympic Association and Swim England, and was even crowned British bodybuilding champion in 1991. Today her USP is cutting through the jargon and translating science into clear and accessible messages to deliver up-to-date, evidence-based information in a practical, accessible way. She's written 28 books on nutrition and fitness, including the best-selling The Complete Guide to Sports Nutrition. *First published in 1993, it is now in its 8th edition, and is recommended reading on many sports nutrition courses. Her most recent titles include* The Vegetarian Athlete's Cookbook *and* Vegetarian Meals in 30 minutes. *Over to Anita to talk you through nutrition approaches for everyday athletes.*

When you start training for long-distance running you can develop a one-track mind. The running is all that matters. It's too easy to forget about the fuel. But you can't have success out on the road and on the trails unless you start thinking about fuel from the start. What you eat, how much you eat and when you eat all combine to impact your performance and your ability to recover. It's also key to your overall health, keeping you free from illness and injury. Fuelling for a race is absolutely a consideration, but this only plays a minuscule part in the journey you'll take from your first training run to the race finish line. Food is what facilitates muscle recovery and physiological adaptations, making you fitter and stronger, all the way through your running journey. When training to lose weight, people can wrongly start to feel like food is the enemy. It's not. When it comes to running, food is your closest ally.

RUN THE NUMBERS

The first thing that you'll need to appreciate when you start running is that your body will need more energy, more calories and more nutrients. It'll need more of absolutely everything. You'll be pleased to know that thinking about food restriction or cutting out certain food categories has no place in a runner's kitchen. That's the number-one rule to remember.

More than that, eating needs to become a priority. That means planning in advance and being organised. You don't need to create a spreadsheet, you don't need to be pedantic, but plan out your week. Know when you're in, know when you're out and it'll help you to have the right things in your kitchen. This way you won't be caught short, resorting to yet another bowl of pesto pasta or grabbing a sandwich on the way back from work.

The meals you plan needn't be complicated and they don't have to be stereotypically bland fitness fuel, either. It helps to think about food in simple categories, understanding what kinds of food fall in those categories and then building a plate of food using the ingredients you like. There is no perfect diet but these are the general guidelines that I recommend.

Think about food in four basic categories:

Fruit and veg
Even the biggest broccoli-phobes know about getting their five a day, but what you've really got to emphasise is the variety of your vegetables. Think about eating a rainbow of colours – red tomatoes, yellow peppers, purple beetroot, green courgettes,

blue blueberries and orange, er, oranges – that way you'll be getting all the vitamins and minerals that can support good health under the stress of a new running plan, plus the fibre and all of the important micronutrients that support the muscle adaptations that make you faster and fitter. Plus, five is good, but chewing your way towards 10 would be even better.

Carbohydrates

Don't *ever* think about cutting out carbohydrates. Ever. Carbs are your muscles' preferred fuel and you can put a great big underline beneath the word preferred because it's important. Carbs are the most efficient fuel because they are easily broken down. They will yield more energy when you're running than other food types and they'll also provide you with that energy more quickly. That will allow you to run faster.

It's true that as the ketogenic diet has transferred across from weird off-shoot to the mainstream that people have researched using fat for fuel during exercise. It does work. But it will only make you a very good slow runner. If you want the ability to run fast then you *need* carbohydrates. Here, of course, we're talking about pasta, rice, quinoa, bread, potatoes and bananas. Again, it pays to make your intake of carbohydrates really varied, emphasising whole grains rather than the more refined and white versions of breads and pasta available. The more natural the better.

Protein

Much like carbs, this has become a contentious macronutrient recently. It's at the centre of the conversation around plant-based diets and athletic performance, for example. But it needn't be complicated. Yes, proteins would come most easily from dairy, meat and fish if they are part of your diet, but if not, these can be substituted for pulses like beans and lentils as well as soy products and nuts. The only difference is that you will need to consume more bulk to hit the recommended target of around 20g per meal, if you want to stimulate maximal muscle recovery and muscle repair after running.

With these ingredients and categories in mind – and at the top of every shopping list from now on – the best way to deploy them at mealtimes is simple. Give them a third of your plate each.

Fats

I count healthy fats as the fourth category, but because they are so calorific the quantities are much smaller. Which is why I believe that it's best to look at building your plate with the three other categories and add a helping of fats as a finishing touch – like the cherry on top of your meal. This could look like: a few flakes of mackerel or avocado with your eggs at breakfast; a few toasted nuts or a glug of olive oil over your salad at lunch.

TOO MUCH OF A GOOD THING

As mentioned, protein is the macro of the moment. Somehow it has transcended its role as nutrient to become a catch-all term for better health. And by somehow I of course mean marketing spiel.

You're led to believe, as a consumer, that you are doing the best possible thing by taking on the most protein possible with every meal. The macro now has a massive health halo and I think it's a backlash from the fat and carb debates. They've been dismissed and demonised, and all that's left is protein, so it has been put on a pedestal. It's a bubble and one that I think will burst fairly soon.

Of course we need protein. It's an essential nutrient that has many, many beneficial effects on the body, but it's not a case of the more the better. You look on social media and protein shakes are everywhere. You can go into a petrol station or corner shop and buy protein-enriched snacks, cereals and even chocolate bars. It's too much. While you need a certain amount, you don't need to over-consume protein and, most importantly, you can absolutely get all the protein you need from whole foods. You don't *need* to have protein supplements. The clue is in the name – they're supplementary and are best used as a safety measure, not a go-to. If you prefer a breakfast of oats and berries it's going to be tough to hit your 20g of protein in that meal, and so that might be the time to stir in some powder. If you're totally slammed at work and only had time to grab a veggie sandwich and a banana, then reaching for the protein bar in your top drawer isn't such a bad idea. They're a good back up, nothing more.

And what's so special about that 20g number? Well, it's just a good guideline of the optimum amount of protein that your body can use for muscle recovery and repair at any one time. It's a myth that if you eat more than 30g your body will just wee it out. But once you go above the amount of protein your body can use, you can't keep on building muscle, so you won't use that protein for muscle synthesis. Instead, it will then be metabolised and broken down and converted into other compounds and used, ultimately, as an energy source in the same way that you would use carbs. So you can eat loads of protein, but that extra grammage is not going to go into your muscles, it won't make you stronger, it won't make your muscles bigger and it won't make you run faster.

Importantly, the trend for going large on protein increases the likelihood that you're *undereating* when it comes to the other major macronutrients. And scrimping on carbs to make way for protein is a major mis-step in a runner's diet.

> **TIP:** If you want to get really scientific then try this: the maximum muscle-building potential of each meal is 0.25g of protein per kilogram of bodyweight. For the average UK woman of 69kg that's 17g.

TIME IT RIGHT

Carbs are your energy source. And it's not just how much you eat, but when you eat them, especially when you're planning on running a race or tackling a high-intensity training session. This is the speed macro. If your carbohydrate stores or blood-sugar levels are low then hitting top gear is impossible. You won't be able to produce energy fast enough and, as a result, you will be a slower runner. You'll find it difficult to accelerate and to run up hills, so it's really important that you don't restrict your carbs, particularly not before those types of session.

The interesting part here, then, is playing with your carb intake depending on the type of day you plan on having. Which, again, is where the meal planning I mentioned earlier comes to the fore. If you have a really big day of running or an active day at work, you'll need to have more food and more carbohydrates. If you don't, you will feel tired, fatigued and recovery will become difficult. Equally, if you are having a lazy day recovering – good for you! – then it makes sense that you consume slightly less food. Don't overthink it, and I don't recommend becoming overly dependent on tracking apps, for example, but instead listen to your body and exercise sense. Move more, eat more. Move less, eat less.

You can drill down further into timings, too. Like, do you

need to time a meal before you run? It's OK to run on an empty stomach if it's a short distance – anything less than an hour and you should manage it fine. In this situation it's down to what you prefer. If you like to run in the mornings, but struggle to eat first thing, that's no problem. However, if you are planning to do your long run, and I'm talking about anything over 60 minutes, then it's absolutely worth your while to eat first.

The best time to eat pre-exercise is about three or four hours beforehand because it gives your body enough time to begin digesting that food and for some of that energy to then go into your bloodstream and be delivered to your muscles. If you eat a big meal too close to your running then you're going to feel uncomfortable and heavy, obviously. It's why I'd recommend saving your long runs for the evenings or weekends if possible.

There are also little tweaks you can make along the way. Let's say you like to train at 6pm and you've had your lunch at 1pm. You've got a gap of five hours and could probably do with a top-up before lacing your trainers. A snack around 30 minutes before your run will help to raise your blood sugar a little and ensure that you're not running hungry, plus it'll help you to keep the intensity up for longer. This principle is truly key when it comes to your Sunday Runday – the traditional time to go after a few extra miles. If you're setting off in the morning, then it's unlikely you're going to rise at 6am on a weekend just to give your breakfast time to digest. This is when you need to fuel properly the day before. Saturday night is really important for getting in your carbs and your protein and making sure that your muscles are filled with glycogen ready to fuel your exertions. That way, when it comes to Sunday morning, you can reach for a banana, a handful of dried fruit or a small bowl of porridge. This will be enough to bump up your blood sugar, see off hunger and make you feel ready to run. All you need is that little kickstart to get you out the door and the stores from Saturday night's pasta dish will take care of the rest.

Crucially, this will also teach you to run with the feeling of having some food inside of you. Not a massive meal, but there's no way you can do a marathon without refuelling, so training is the time – especially on those long runs – to get used to running with something in your stomach.

EATING ON THE GO

Eating (or fuelling) during a run comes into play on any run longer than about an hour. Between 60 and 90 minutes is a crucial period because that's when your glycogen stores (the energy in your muscles and your liver) start to deplete and fatigue sets in. You'll have to slow down your pace or you may need to stop altogether. You need to start refuelling before you hit rock bottom. If you're new to running and pounding your local park at a steady pace, then the best time to do this is around 45–60 minutes, although this depends on how hard you're pushing and how well you stocked up the night before.

The types of foods you take with you are also crucial. This is where everything you know about nutrition is inverted. You don't need to be having complex, nutrient-dense foods when you're out running. You're after simple carbs and that means sugar. Yes, sugar. It's not good for your teeth, but it's actually really beneficial to your performance because it is absorbed fast, gets into your blood fast and to your muscles fast. This will allow you to keep going for longer at your chosen pace.

The type of real foods that I recommend would be bananas. You could also try dates or other dried fruit. I like making my own homemade versions of energy bars and balls. They're simple and work out cheaper than the stuff you're reaching for in Whole Foods. All you need to do is pour a mixture of dried fruit and nuts into a food processor, blitz them and roll them into balls. But if you're not sold on that, Jelly Babies also work . . .

And gels? Well, they're heavily promoted and it's easy for runners to think that they need them. You don't. The benefits are that you know you're going to get an exact amount of carbohydrate in one sachet and they're easy to slip into the pocket of your running backpack. But there's nothing fancy or scientific about them. They're just sugars and there are, I would suggest, better ways to get those sugars that are, crucially, easier on your digestion.

Because gels are so concentrated they can be quite gloopy and don't sit well in everyone's stomachs. Some people love them, some people hate them. Fuelling *during* a run is probably the most individual part of a nutrition plan for runners. It's something, really, that you need to work out for yourself. That means practising. Now. I would suggest starting small – with a single bite of banana, say – and build up gradually. Real food will be kinder to your stomach to begin with, but if you feel like you need a bigger hit then by all means try a gel.

However, what you'll find when you've been running for a long time is that things can slow down in the upper part of your gut and speed up in the bottom. And that's a recipe for disaster. A gel can go in and, well, come out again pretty much immediately. It does happen to an awful lot of runners and it's why you need to be testing out gels weeks before race day.

MAKING THE CUT

Having sugar as your major ally can be problematic. It's not uncommon today for people to have cut it out completely. However, if you're serious about running long distances then you *need* it. It worries me that so many people, including runners, are adopting these restrictive food practices for no good reason. Of course you know sugar is not good for your teeth, and scoffing Krispy Kremes every night on the sofa will wreck your health, but that doesn't mean that we've got to ban all types of sugar, especially if we're active. The most worrying thing is when people cut out fruit and dried fruit. There is no science whatsoever to support the benefits of cutting out perfectly good snacks like these, you've just got to put everything into perspective. Eat dates by the fistful and of course it's going to become problematic, as with most other food. However, once you start putting bans in place and start restricting yourself, that's going to harm your mental health.

I see very many cases of orthorexia, where people become obsessed with trying to eat the right things all the time. They may achieve their goal of losing weight in the short term, but can create a really unhealthy scenario in both their mental and physical health after time.

And that's another interesting conundrum that comes with running. Plenty of people take up running or sign up to the marathon to lose weight, but it doesn't happen. Some people find that they even get heavier. It's even got a name – marathon weight gain. People assume that something happens to their metabolism, that the body alters physiologically and that results in them gaining weight. I'm afraid that's not true at all. The reasons are far more prosaic.

Firstly, when you start running you feel really exhausted even after the first kilometre. You're therefore warranted to think, 'Oh, I've run so much, I must have burned through so many calories.' It's therefore easy to overestimate your burn rate and treat yourself afterwards, or think that you can then relax your eating plan for the rest of the day. The problem is, that the 300kcals you worked so hard to burn off are almost entirely offset by a single Snickers bar. Secondly, you experience an increase in appetite when you first begin running and it therefore becomes easy to eat more than intended. Combine these factors and it's not hard to see why you're no longer in the calorie deficit you need to lose weight. However, let me give you some reassurance that if you're running regularly your appetite will right itself.

It's also really important to say that you do not have to be skinny; you don't have to be built like Mo Farah to be a great runner. There's no perfect running weight that's right for everyone. You've got to run at the weight that's right for you. Running is about improving your health and letting weight become the driving factor can compromise that physically, but also mentally.

DIGGING FOR VICTORY

One in three people has either reduced or cut out meat completely. And it's become very popular among athletes, for example: Lewis Hamilton the F1 driver, Tom Daley the diver and Adam Peaty the Olympic swimmer. But one area where it has become particularly popular is among distance runners.

There are a variety of reasons why people are now choosing to adopt a plant-based approach. In the latest report, nearly half of the respondents cited 'health' as the number-one reason for their dietary switch. The other main reasons are weight management – not that I think that's necessarily a good reason – and then concern over animal welfare, environment and sustainability, which were leading factors particularly among under 35s. When it comes to health we know from population studies that people who follow a plant-based diet or a vegetarian or vegan diet have a significantly lower risk of cardiovascular disease and certain cancers.

But there is another aspect, and that relates to performance. Despite it being adopted by athletes more and more, there are still misconceptions that swapping to being plant-based will make supporting and fuelling athletic performance more difficult. But that's not the case. A big review by Australian researchers in 2016[19] concluded there is no disadvantage to cutting out meat.

In fact, there was a separate Arizona State University study in 2017[20] that compared the performance of vegetarians and meat eaters and found no difference in the men, but for women there was actually an improvement among the vegetarians. They had a higher level of cardio-respiratory fitness compared to those who ate meat. Which is obviously good news for runners.

As I mentioned earlier, for so long we've been fed the notion that it's hard to eat enough protein on a plant-based diet. This is a myth. You can absolutely get enough to fuel performance as a vegetarian or vegan. There are many, many sources and they come in two categories: complete proteins, which contain all of the essential amino acids (though they are few and far between, the main ones being hemp and soya) and incomplete proteins, which don't contain the entire amino-acid profile.

The key, therefore, is to introduce variety. If you're a vegetarian then you can lean heavily on dairy and eggs, or if you are completely vegan then you can reach for pulses, nuts and seeds as your go-tos. The key is to layer in protein-rich foods throughout the day – spreading some peanut butter on toast in the morning won't be enough. If you're having a chickpea and spinach curry, for example, your chickpeas have protein, but then I would serve it with a grain and probably stir in some cashews. That's a simple way to layer in a variety of incomplete proteins to ensure you get a complete set of amino acids at dinner time.

Your vegan shopping list for protein:

- Tofu
- Hemp seed
- Flaxseed
- Nuts
- Nut butters
- Beans
- Lentils
- Quinoa

MICRO MANAGEMENT FOR VEGANS

When swapping to veganism you do run the risk of certain deficiencies, but there are simple ways to cover all bases.

Omega-3
This mainly comes from oily fish. The best wholefood sources for vegans are seeds and walnuts. However, you'd need to be eating at least a tablespoonful per day, which may be a struggle for even the most committed walnut eater. In these cases, there are alternative vegetarian omega-3 supplements based on algae oil.

Calcium

Cutting out dairy can make topping up this micro difficult. Tofu is a good source, but soya milk and almond milk are now fortified with calcium, so be liberal pouring them over your morning muesli.

Vitamin B12

You can't get this from traditional plant sources, and if your levels drop you run the risk of anaemia, which will impact your energy levels and cause fatigue, particularly during exercise. The fortified plant milks offer a decent dose, as does Marmite. If you're taking a multivitamin, this will also be enough – there's no need for an individual supplement.

Iron

Meat is a rich source of this energy-supporting micronutrient, but you can also easily get enough from nuts, beans, lentils and whole grains. Again, you just need to eat a variety of ingredients. If you struggle to do this, or feel your energy levels flagging, then a good tip to remember is to have a source of vitamin C (abundant in fruits and vegetables) at the same time as iron-rich foods to increase absorption.

WHAT'S COOKING?

The most common concern about healthy cooking and sticking to your plan as a runner is that food prep can be complicated and time-consuming. But there are ways around this. One-pot meals make life easy in the kitchen. There's not much washing up and you can make batches that last the week with anything left over being frozen for the times that you're caught short in the future. You don't need to have any special cooking techniques, either. Follow the ingredient guidelines above, stick it all in a pot, *et voilà*! OK, that's not strictly true, but you can make a start by following the recipe overleaf and go from there.

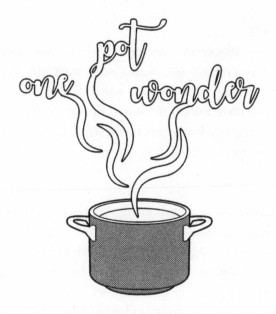

Meal prep with my one-pot Chickpea and Spinach Curry from my book *The Runner's Cookbook*

Packed with protein, fibre, iron and vitamin C, this is one of my go-to meals when I'm short on time and my fridge is practically empty. The best thing about this recipe is that it can be assembled almost entirely from store-cupboard ingredients (if you use frozen rather than fresh spinach) and requires very little chopping!

SERVES 4
1 tbsp light olive oil or rapeseed oil
1 onion, chopped
3–4 garlic cloves, crushed
2.5cm piece of fresh ginger, peeled and finely grated
½ red chilli (or to taste), finely chopped
2 tbsp mild curry paste (or to taste)
1 x 400g tin of chopped tomatoes
2 x 400g tins of chickpeas, drained and rinsed
200ml hot water
200g fresh or frozen spinach
A handful of fresh coriander leaves, chopped
Squeeze of lemon juice
Salt and freshly ground black pepper

To serve: whole-grain rice and Greek yogurt

Heat the oil in a large heavy-based saucepan over a medium heat, add the onion and fry over a moderate heat for 5 minutes until translucent. Add the garlic, ginger, chilli and curry paste. Cook for a further minute.

Add the tomatoes, chickpeas and hot water. Bring to the boil, then simmer for 10 minutes. Add the spinach and stir until the spinach has wilted. Remove from the heat, season with salt and pepper, and stir in the fresh coriander and lemon juice. Serve with the rice and Greek yogurt.

Per serving (without rice): 263kcal, 17g protein, 8g fat (1g saturates), 26g carbs (7g total sugars), 9g fibre

On The Run With . . . Hannah Fields

Hannah Fields is a middle-distance running star and seven-time NAIA champion in the USA. It's her job to run well and fuel right. However, on 26 June 2018 she revealed to the world that she was also fighting a running battle with an eating disorder. It's an issue that is surprisingly prevalent in female distance running. In 2007, researchers at the Norwegian School of Sports Sciences[21] found that about 47 per cent of elite female athletes in sports that 'emphasised leanness' (of which running is one) had clinically diagnosed eating disorders compared with 21 per cent of women in the general population. She's walking proof that these diseases do not discriminate and that, just because you know something is harmful doesn't mean you will be able to resist it. She has since taken the inspirational route to be open and honest about her difficulties and chart her path to recovery. Here I try to keep up as we discuss her journey, the often troublesome relationship between food and exercise, and making sure that everyone knows that life will have its ups, downs, setbacks and successes – and that's very much OK.

AL: It's a brave step to share a story so personal as an eating disorder, but you have made a point of taking that a step further. In your revelatory Instagram post you said you wanted to be open before you became a 'success story'. Why do you feel it was important to make that distinction?

HF: When I originally decided to seek out treatment those thoughts weren't going through my head at all. I was in such a dark place, I had no other options but to seek out help. It wasn't until a month into intensive treatment that I realised I could provide a frame of reference for other people who are struggling with it.

As someone who's experiencing it in the midst of it [an eating disorder], it's confusing. You want to know what to expect. But you have to let go of those expectations because this isn't going to be linear. It isn't easy, and I realised there's no particular way that this issue is meant to look. And so, in coming to terms with that I then realised that I could have this cool opportunity to share what I'm battling as I go through it.

But that wasn't my initial concern. I wanted to be in a place where I felt confident that sharing wasn't going to derail my own recovery. Being a person that people look to to be their sense of security is a responsibility. I spoke to my therapist before doing it and they said, 'I want to support you but I want you to be motivated from a place of love and not obligation.'

AL: What was going on in the run-up to you realising you had a problem? Was there a specific moment where you decided that you wanted to take action, or was it something that crept up on you gradually?

HF: It was kind of both. There was a lot of building up to this breaking moment. I had had a relatively successful track season the previous year and I had worked so hard to attain that; my whole world centred around it, my whole identity centred around it. I desperately wanted to hold onto it. Ironically, however, the way I was coping with that was in a harmful way and I was only going to sabotage my chances of running success. It gradually led to eating-disorder behaviours (bingeing and purging), becoming part of my life – all done in secret.

The hiddenness of all of that was eating me inside out – no pun intended! I wasn't living in accordance with who I wanted to be, and it was impacting on my love for the sport and my relationships, too. But then the breaking point came. It was right before we were supposed to do a long stint at altitude and I was going to be away for four to six weeks. The pressure of being away from home and dealing with this overwhelmed me. I just broke down and told my husband that I needed serious help. I couldn't go away for a month and not have the support around me that I needed.

I called my coach and eventually I was able to share with my teammates as well. Beautifully, everyone was supportive in realising that my health was the priority.

AL: The fact that it is an illness is obviously what makes this so sad, but I am interested to get an insight into the battle that must have been playing out inside your head. As a sportswoman you would have had an understanding of the impact that nutrition has on performance, yet food became a central problem in your day-to-day. Can you explain the thoughts that you were dealing with?

HF: I wish I could perfectly answer that question. I can't speak for everyone, but a lot of people do things that they know aren't helpful. I and others do things that I know are hurtful. It makes no logical sense. But what I've learned, and am still trying to learn as a life-long process, is that because my identity was wrapped around running, and my performance, and how I was viewed according to my performances, I felt so out of control. I did, however, feel a sense of control in this little area with food.

The strange thing is that this eventually led to not being in control at all. I think that was one of the hardest things about sharing. I was trying to articulate these things that – if I were to have no political correctness about – you would easily say are so stupid. It makes no sense at all. If these are your goals and desires, whether it's running or anything, it doesn't even have to be sport, this isn't helpful. But that's what makes it a mental illness.

AL: That issue of control is interesting because that isn't specific to professional runners. It can be someone running to lose weight, or someone running to offset the stresses of work. That relationship between food and exercise is so crucial. How did it affect your training?

HF: When it was at its peak, about a year and a half ago, it was like every run, every race, every workout, I felt like I was drained. I had no energy.

AL: I'm guessing both mentally and physically . . .

HF: Yes. I couldn't draw a line between the two. It was just a total sense of fatigue. It wasn't always connected to my weight, either. It wasn't like the peak of my disorder was my lowest weight. There's no correlation there. It was just what was going on internally. It really derailed my training. And also, as anybody who is getting into running will know, you have disappointing workouts, and you have periods of time where you're fatigued, and that can be discouraging as well. And that started a cycle of beating down my confidence, which only served to make things worse.

AL: In contrast, talk to me about the recovery process. How is it manifesting itself, what advice are you being given, what steps are you taking in terms of food?

HF: It evolved over time. I've been told that my relationship with food is going to evolve as I build my fundamentals again;

what it feels like to be full and what it feels like to have hunger temptations. It might sound silly to someone who's never experienced this before but, for me at least, I had operated according to the guidelines I set for myself. I would only eat certain amounts and anything more was outside of the rules. But then sometimes I would overindulge and push myself way past the point of fullness, which caused the bingeing and purging cycle.

All the biological components of hunger and fullness were totally out of whack, because I didn't trust my body. So I started this rebuilding phase of eating according to my body's needs and understanding what that feels like. And then, as I progressed through the treatment centre, I was able to implement more training.

AL: So you've been trying to get back to a form of intuitive eating?

HF: Exactly, I had to relearn it. It sounds crazy because that's what we're born with. Babies know when they're hungry, they know when they're full. So that was the biggest piece of learning, that intuition. Once I did that, I was able to progress to become more prescriptive with my nutrition. Which means, as an athlete, knowing I've got to get a certain amount of protein and carbohydrates after running to refuel.

The key is learning what's a healthy way of doing that, and what's an obsessive and unhealthy way of doing that. That was tricky. It's been really helpful to have a dietician that I work with to give that accountability. Having someone that I'm accountable to and who's aware of what's going on. They're not tracking every mouthful but I have a relationship with them where if things start to go amiss then I have help to fill in the gaps.

AL: It's wonderful that you're making so much progress. When you're going through a good period, when you feel like you're eating what your body needs, you've got your mindset in the right place – how does that cross over to boost your training?

HF: Completely. I sleep better, I recover better. And running is enjoyable in the way that it's meant to be. It's a gift and when I'm in a good place I'm running as a way to fulfil that potential, not as a means for justification, like I have to be validated through my running. When all those pieces are in harmony, the running falls into place without me having to grip so tightly.

AL: Since you opened up on Instagram, can you talk me through people's reactions?

HF: I was really humbled by how much positivity came out of it and that I saw zero negative responses. Everyone was extremely supportive. Every week I get new people reaching out to me, sharing their experiences about how my story has empowered them to seek treatment, or to start the process of working out 'how do I get help,' even when they're not ready to ask for it quite yet.

That has been really encouraging for me as well, to just be held accountable in my own recovery. I feel a sense of responsibility, and not in a negative way. I want to continue down this path because I want other people to know it's possible. Real recovery is possible.

AL: You said you don't want to be seen as a success story because you're not done. But can I ask, do you feel you're going to become one in the end?

HF: I want to say yes. I don't want to downplay the fact that I could. But most importantly, I also don't want to see success as never relapsing. I'm holding the term 'success story' kind of loosely. Success to me would be continuing to be vulnerable but continuing to move forward and allow myself more freedom.

I still feel ashamed and I wish this wasn't a part of my story – I really do. But equally I'm not letting it define me and plan on using it for good. I can't change the fact that I have this thorn in my flesh and I have to continue to walk with humility and grace about it. And I'm not naturally drawn to social media, I'm just more of a private person, but there is good that can come from this and I want to realise that.

AL: What words of advice would you give to people who are in the midst of it now, or perhaps feel themselves slipping in the wrong direction?

HF: The first part is to recognise that something isn't right and that the issue may be greater than you want to admit. But then to be gracious with yourself and to be kind. Put yourself in someone else's shoes and react to yourself as you would to someone who opened up with these issues to you. How would you respond to someone who came to you for help? Realise that it's OK to have these battles.

Then share with someone that you trust and who has your best interests in mind. That may be with a professional, or if that feels like a little bit too big of a step, then with someone that you trust.

There are so many little steps along the way. They're going to be backwards, forwards, sideways, so you cannot look at this like 'I have an eating disorder, I need to go into treatment or go to a hospital'; take little steps.

We had this picture on the wall at my treatment centre. It was an upwards line and then a super-messy squiggle in the middle and an upwards line to end. That is what recovery looks like.

There really is hope. This is a painful thing to experience and I wouldn't wish it on anyone, but I think the things in our life that hurt and are hard and make us want to hide, they are things that really strenghten us. And that makes me smile, it makes me have joy, and be able to accept the cards that I have been dealt. I accept that this is something I've battled but it's also turned me into the person that I think I'm meant to be. There's so much good that can come out of this and knowing that can wipe away a lot of the fear that comes with the words 'eating disorder'.

> **Your Chapter 4 Action Plan**
>
> • Realise that food is your greatest ally in running, and carbs are king! (Or kween!)
>
> • A third of your plate should be given to protein, carbs and veg with a dollop of fat on top
>
> • Time your carbs right. If you're running early, stock up on energy the night before
>
> • Start practising with your mid-run fuel now. And remember, energy gels can backfire – if you know what I mean . . .
>
> • Master the one-pot recipe and batch-cook your way to fuelling success

CHAPTER 5

Weights Off Your Mind

My Journey

Like many women I'd always felt uncomfortable in the weights room at the gym. It was the domain of pumped-up bros in string vests, equally likely to offer you their phone number as unwanted form advice. But it pays to be strong and claim your own space among the barbells. This is how heavy metal finally made me feel like a real runner.

What if I told you that you could get better at running by running less? Would you believe me? Thousands wouldn't, I'm sure. Perhaps it's because we're conditioned to believe that more means more. More work means more success. More training runs mean more successful run times. Or maybe it's because, since school, we've been led to believe that running is a simple case of putting one foot in front of the other – albeit quickly. Some people are slow, others are quick, but remember kids, 'Practice makes perfect!' And so off we go, out on yet another run, thinking that's the only way we're going to get faster. But we've had it all wrong.

At no point during my school years, taking part in a non-negotiable, soggy cross-country, or sweating through a baking-hot 200m on sports day, was I told to activate my glutes. Nor did my mum get me to do single-legged step-ups on the patio before encouraging me to wobble as fast as I could to the end of the garden while learning to walk. Perhaps if she did, I might have made it a few more strides before face-planting the flowerbed. That's because, knowing what I know now, I'm well aware that boosting strength is the true key to supercharging your stride.

(Side note: I fear for my unborn children, too. I'm pretty sure Future Me will have them doing core activations at soft play. Sorry, kids.)

But really, running well today involves more than just running, and my first marathon journey was testament to that.

NOT FEELING GOOD ENOUGH

In 2011 I ran a half marathon with three generations of my family. For months I'd text my nan to compare our training notes as we edged closer to the Run to the Beat start line. And those notes brought us all closer together as a family; during those 12 weeks, race chat replaced small talk and all three generations formed a bond.

Fast-forward a few years and I'd been sucked in to the fitness bubble. Every day I lived and breathed fitness culture, both IRL and virtually, and took great satisfaction in adding to that conversation via my own social-media account. However, I was unaware of what this deification of fitness was doing to my mental health. It's said that people with bulimia often have perfectionist tendencies and that they can feel inadequate in some way or have a strong desire to gain approval of others – had I known this, and not been in denial about my eating disorder, then I would have thought twice about joining social media. But I didn't and I did.

And so, unbeknown to me, my mind started to pitch my personal fitness progress against those getting thousands of double-taps. My head became a whirring mess of constant thoughts surrounding the perfect self-image and the ideal body-weight. These toxic emotions spilled over into other areas of my life too.

In fact, for the first year or so of working at *Women's Health* I was sure someone was going to tap me on my shoulder and say, 'Sorry, we made a mistake in the interview process and you're out.' Every day I couldn't believe that they'd chosen me ahead of the other candidates and my response was to hustle harder than I'd ever hustled before.

No longer could anything I worked on be just 'OK' – it had to be perfect. It had to be up to the same standard as the content that graced the pages of the magazine, which was winning awards as the UK's most successful women's magazine of the decade. But then the lines between my work life and my personal one started to blur. The extreme ideals I placed on my work, I started to place upon myself. No longer could I just be good at something, I had to be in the elite. I wanted to be among the fittest in the office and on Instagram. When it came to the gym, I got pretty damn good – there's a reason I have the bio line 'I can't dance but I can burpee'. However, when it came to running I just couldn't keep up. I couldn't break a sub-25-minute 5k, or get close to a 45-minute 10k. I wasn't as fast as the 'real runners' – those who ran a 5k on their lunch break in the same time it took me to get my quinoa salad from the shop 400m down the road.

And so, because I wasn't a runner I gravitated towards the fitness that I was good at. I went to every fitness-class launch in London and pushed myself through the infamous but gruelling Bikini Body Guide workouts on lunch. But it turns out you really can have too much of a good thing. My fixation with HIIT led to burnout. It was this fitness downfall, however, that led to the most important plot twist in my running journey. By forcing me to slow down, redirecting me from the HIIT class to the weights room, it afforded me the opportunity to learn how to lift. Here I discovered that becoming strong in body and mind is the perfect foundation to build a runner's body, and it's something that I wish more women knew.

According to Sport England, 13 million women would like to participate more in sport and physical activity.[22] Of these women, nearly half do no exercise at all. That's the same as the whole population of Denmark doing less than 30 minutes of activity a week. That's 6 million women not even walking 4 minutes a day – a stat I often struggle to compute. But at other times, it's also something I empathise with. If I, a health editor who has regularly engaged with fitness since my teens, is plagued by run-timidation, then I can see why the 57 per cent of UK females who are classified as either overweight or obese can feel alienated in the age of #fitspo. Add in the fact that running with extra weight puts increased pressure and stress on the bones and joints, particularly in the lower back, causing aches and pains, then it's easy to see why more than twice as many UK adults avoid running at all costs.

Feeling anxious over fitness doesn't discriminate. I still remember being surprised by Ellie Goulding's admission that she too can feel like an imposter when working out: 'I'll run up and down [at my local gym] and not a lot of women do that,' she told *Women's Health.* 'I don't want to draw attention to myself at the best of times, but at the gym men stop what they're doing and look at you with a smug smile that bums me out so much. But I won't stop. I won't stop running up and down just because they're staring at me as if what I'm doing is out of the ordinary or unladylike. F*** that.'

This only adds to the argument that we need to get comfortable with feeling uncomfortable if we are to succeed at our goals. However, that doesn't mean subscribing to tired notions about 'running to get fit', and in doing so that you have to endure endless, boring slogs of pounding pavements. That's as outdated as the tired pair of Asics gathering dust in your cupboard. Today, it's all about getting *fit to run*. And the weights room is where I laid the physical and mental foundations to outmuscle intimidation and feelings of inadequacy and built the strength to run well far.

STRENGTH TO STRENGTH

The crossover benefits of flexing my new muscles to flexing on my mile times came to fruition in 2017. In the year leading up to then I'd spent four days a week learning how to lift. I'll never forget the day that I ripped an Olympic bar weighing more than my bodyweight up from the floor. As I held the steel bar in front of my crotch I finally knew what people mean by Big Dick Energy. The confidence that I had as a child, that had been bashed out of me during my first years struggling in London, was back. I didn't need to shout about my achievement because staring back in the mirror was 58kg me holding all 93kg of the bar and *damn* did it feel good. It was the way weights made me feel that had me returning to the barbell again and again.

It was during this time that, after a particularly unfortunate bob haircut, my husband (through suppressed laughter) told me I looked like He Man. Now, he has since told me that it was to do with the hair, but I panicked, thinking that he was calling me out for being bulky. The fear that weights will turn you into a beast is a common one, but it's unfounded. (Not that there's anything wrong with biceps on a woman – I'm in awe of CrossFitter Sara Sigmundsdóttir every time I rewatch the CrossFit documentaries on Netflix!) And, yes, at this time I was certainly strong, but if I really wanted to be built like a superhero I would have to do far more than lift weights. You see, women don't have nearly as much testosterone as men, which makes packing on big shoulders more difficult. Plus, you need a hefty calorie surplus in your diet to add size, so as long you're keeping an eye on your food, there's no reason for weightlifting to change the way you look. It will, however, change the way you *feel* – especially when running.

It's strength that can help you to get better at running by running less. When I started marathon training I was strong. And by being strong, I was fast. My times were minutes quicker than earlier in my 20s and I finally started to feel like those 'real runners'. But speed wasn't the only benefit. It's no secret that running training – especially for a marathon – is an exercise in endurance, and that refers to far more than just how much puff you have. Strength gives your body endurance and gives you the physical grit you need to keep going. And, if you're lucky, stay injury-free.

PREHAB NOT REHAB

Over the years, plenty of research has been done to link injury rates in runners with the types of training variables that we're in control of. For example, volume, distance, duration, frequency, intensity and speed. We all get to decide how much or little we do and how fast we're going to run. One review of more than 4,500 research papers[23] shone the spotlight on a particularly interesting statistic: the annual injury rate for runners can be as high as 85 per cent. That's nearly 9 out of every 10 runners being relegated to the physio table, which can get expensive. The average session can cost runners £40–60 a pop to get them back up and running.

Lifting weights, or strength training to some, is a crucial ally in stopping yourself becoming part of that statistic. It builds a stronger, more robust structure, and this functional training add-on can help to counteract all the wear and tear of running. At times during my marathon training I was hitting nearly 50 miles a week. That's a hell of a lot of jumping from one foot to the other, yet I never once pulled a muscle or had to pull out of a training run. The same can't be said for other runners that I know who have been frog-marched to the gym by physios and osteopaths when it's too late. By then they're undoing damage, rather than preventing it.

Over the course of training for my first marathon, I cut my gym sessions from four to two a week, but in that time I maintained the strength needed to withstand the physical battering of marathon training, and the lower-body power that ensured, come race day, my muscles were ready.

On the day, in the last half-mile when I was crying behind my sunglasses and running on crowd enthusiasm and not much else, I doubted that my body had anything left in it except the farts caused by one-too-many energy gels. However, as I came around the corner by Buckingham Palace I remembered those gym sessions. I thought about the hours spent in the corner of Third Space gym telling myself to believe in my body as I sprang from the floor up on to the plyo box in front of me. I remembered the sessions on the TRX when I tried desperately not to topple over. I conjured up the memory of lunging up and down the gym track moaning about getting big quads. Then, as I saw a runner dressed as a giant poo emoji make a dash for the finish line, I did too. My legs suddenly picked up pace. I could feel my glutes firing and my arms pumping – I was chasing down the giant poo. In fact, I was nearly overtaking the giant poo. The crowds were cheering and so was my inner cheerleader. After nearly four hours of running I was now in touching distance of the big Virgin Money banners and about to cross under the race clock. I got faster and faster, closer and closer, and then it happened. I sprinted across the finish line and became a champion – and a champion of strength training to boot.

The *Journal of Sports Sciences* confirmed the benefits of weights for running nearly a decade ago,[24] but the uptake, especially in women, has been painfully slow. If you really want to get ahead of the pack then you need to take a few days off running and give your performance a lift. Do it and maybe you too could be immortalised on the BBC overtaking a giant poo emoji on the way to marathon glory.

'Workouts don't get easier, you get stronger'

Follow The Leader

Luke Worthington is an expert sports scientist and Nike trainer who has a wealth of experience in elite level sport. He's also got a very cute dog called Bob, but that's less relevant. He specialises in biomechanics and is the very best at what he does – chiefly, getting celebrities, runners and everyday athletes to train hard but well. It's what makes him one of the most sought-after trainers in the country. Luke is also the guy who has got me around two marathons, plus a number of half marathons, injury-free and stronger and faster than ever. And now here he is to share that expertise with you.

GETTING FROM A TO B

Getting out and going for a run is worthy. There's no denying that. Whether it's to clear your head before a tough day at work, or simply to move your body after eight hours hunched over a desk, it works. But, when it comes to performance, aimless workouts and runs garner aimless results. That too is undeniable.

If you want to start moving forward, the first thing you need to do is work out where you are and where you want to go. It sounds silly, but the first part of making a training plan is having a plan. You'd be surprised by how many people start their 'fitness journey' without having any idea of where it's going. Around January time, people can start for the sake of it, because it's the done thing, and then they wonder why it doesn't stick past February.

You need a point A and a point B for long-term success. And it doesn't matter what point B is. It doesn't have to be a grand, wholesome ambition to be worthwhile. Yes, it could be running your first marathon. Equally, it could be committing to a Parkrun streak. However, deciding on what your point B is is the easy part. Understanding your point A, on the other hand, is infinitely more important and a little more difficult to nail down.

If you can, getting assessed is super important. If you have access to a qualified and experienced trainer who's got some kind of background in biomechanics then they'll provide you with an invaluable idea of where you're starting out. If you can't do this, then there are plenty of very good amateur athletics clubs, track clubs and running groups that will have coaches able to help you to understand where your starting point is. You just need to ask.

Give yourself an understanding of your starting point in terms of your overall fitness, technical ability and movement ability, then you've got a fighting chance of getting to point B.

WHAT THE HELL IS BIOMECHANICS?

Wake up! Don't drift off just yet, please. Biomechanics is working out the nitty gritty of your body, and not just saying 'sod it' and going for a run. Understanding it will make any cardio endeavour more enjoyable and more successful over time.

Simply put, biomechanics is the science of human movement. Beyond that dictionary definition, what it really means is looking under the bonnet of how somebody does a particular task. How are you sitting on your chair at the moment? How might you then stand up? And how will you walk up the stairs? It's having an understanding of how your body moves and then – even though there are idiosyncrasies between individuals, of course – it's about realising how you *should* be moving and working out how to get there.

The human body has evolved to move in a particular way to avoid excessive wear and tear on any one part. It should therefore move in a balanced, reciprocal way. When it doesn't, that's when you get into trouble. Think about your car, for example. If one wheel gets out of alignment, that tyre will wear down more quickly. The same is true of your body. Imbalances will hurt. But they're also very common – it's why so many people can refer to their 'bad knee' or 'sore shoulder'. The body is incredibly robust and, in the most part, it can handle much of what we ask of it, but it can break down and there is invariably a mechanical explanation behind it; much like with your car, thankfully it can be fixed. And that's why you need the whole picture. You need to work with a coach, or understand yourself, how your own body moves and how it should move. Then you can plot a course to align the two.

The problem comes when people are impatient. It's a running plan, after all. People wonder when the hell are they going to get running?! But allow me to explain why, especially with runners, this is so important. You're not just doing the movements of running once or twice. If you've got to fix the biomechanics of a deadlift, at least you're only doing three sets of 10 reps. When you're training for and running a race, for example, you're doing tens of thousands of the same imbalanced reps over and again.

And so, when it gets to the business end of your long runs – two or three hours in – you're doing everything under extreme mental, physical and emotional fatigue. That's when technique starts to break down. The last thing on your mind is focusing on where your shoulders are, whether your jaw is relaxed or how you're swinging your arms. Instead, it's screaming, 'Get me to the end!' and 'Where's the rosé?'

So, what we have to think of – before we get to this point

– is imprinting mechanically sound and strong movement in these early stages of your training. That way, when you're reaching for the end of your race, you can hang on. And that's where the gym comes in. You need to get fit to run, not immediately focus on running to get fit.

FIT TO RUN

Don't be fooled by the physical stereotypes of long-distance runners as long-legged waifs. If you want to be a runner, you need to be strong. I talk a lot about people 'bullet-proofing' themselves in this early stage of training. And this is done specifically in the gym to supplement the work they're doing on the road.

The slow 'n' steady approach to running on the road that I recommend will gradually build up your capacity for distance and your fitness levels. In addition, what you do in the gym helps your body to become resilient enough to cope with the demands of running. And if that sounds complicated, don't worry, it's not.

When I teach at seminars and I ask trainers how many movements you can do, I get varied answers: 400? 10,000? A million?! And they're right. But they're also wrong. They're right in that there are an unlimited number of variations that you can do, but fundamentally there are just four – and that's where you need to start.

All you need to do is focus on these four movements:

- Squats
- Hinges
- Pushes
- Pulls

Do these and you're on the path to greatness.

For the nerds among you, allow me to break it down a little further.

Squat

This is when you have two feet on the floor and your hips going up and down.

Hinge

This is two feet on the floor and your hips going back and forward. A deadlift is a common example.

(Note: you've got single-leg variations of both a squat and a hinge, so single-leg squats, which are your lunges, and single-leg deadlifts which are, well, exactly as they sound.)

Pushes + pulls

A press-up and a pull-up are good examples of push and pull movements. The variations here normally focus on direction. So, a press-up is a horizontal push, a pull-up is a vertical pull, and then a cable row is a horizontal pull, and pushing something above your head is a vertical push.

When you're sifting through all of the workout content available on the internet – some of which is good and some of which is very, very bad – keep these four movements in mind. Do the moves the workout plan suggests fit easily into these categories? If they do, great. If they don't and instead they look weird and promise to target your 'outer booty' or 'lower six-pack', then steer well clear.

The good thing about running is that it's simple. Effectively you're following a single-leg hinge pattern on each leg, one after the other, over and over again. Which may help you to understand (and make you feel better about!) why running is so bloody tiring. Take me, for example – I weigh 100 kilos, so in order for me to run I've got to propel 100 kilos through the air from one foot. Then I've got to land on another foot and absorb those 100 kilos, plus the momentum, without damaging myself. Having absorbed that force I've then got to reverse it and propel it the other way, back to the first foot. And that's only my first two strides. It's a lot of force to produce and then absorb over and over and over and over again, which provides a cast-iron case for building strength in the gym before you go hammer and tongs pounding the pavements.

MAKE YOUR MOVES

One of the first ports of call for any person I'm training to do a long-distance race is to master the deadlift. Frustratingly, that sounds very masculine, gym-bro-y and, well, off-putting to many women getting fit to run, but it shouldn't. Women have equal place in (and get just as much out of) the weights room as men.

You need to learn how to produce force with your hips, using those hinge movements I mentioned under load, so that you can become strong enough to propel your bodyweight. Secondly, you then need to practise it while you're fatigued so that you can cope with that movement at the end of your run. When I trained Amy for her first marathon I would do something similar to test her strength when she was tired. That would often involve putting her through a miserable few sets on the VersaClimber machine to exhaust her, but then, rather than let her collapse on the floor to recover, I'd ask her to grab a couple of dumbbells and start stepping up on to a box. She'd have to focus on keeping good posture, staying strong in her core and contracting through her glutes to get her up there. She swore at me a lot. But these were all the lessons she needed in her head to stay strong when the going got tough on marathon day.

And so, as mentioned, these basic moves: squats, deadlifts, pull-ups and chest presses should be the basis of your initial training plan for the first four weeks, at least. And you should work heavy, focusing on low reps and lots of rest. You don't need to be out of breath – at this stage your time in the gym is about building strength, not making yourself pour with sweat. You can do that later out on the road.

A good workout is not necessarily a sweaty workout. And that's part of the problem many people have – they're impatient. Doing these workouts three times a week can, admittedly, numb the brain and when you're busy trying to squeeze sessions into a busy schedule, then a sweaty HIIT session can feel like a more effective workout. It isn't. Stick with the barbells for a month and you'll begin to outmuscle fatigue on your longer runs and your training on the road will become far more enjoyable. Strength work is there to complement your runs, not to make you so sore that you can't do them.

The next thing to consider is how much time do you have to hit the gym? There's little point in choosing a three-day-a-week strength programme if you only have time for two sessions. Talking of two sessions a week, this is an example runner's gym plan that only requires two hours a week of commitment.

Note: each phase is 4 weeks. Complete 3 sets of 8 reps for each move (that's 8 on each if it's single leg) but if you're struggling on the squats or deadlifts, move the rep count down to 6.

	Day 1	Day 2
Phase 1 (Fundamentals)	Goblet squat Single-leg RDL TRX hamstring curl TRX rollout	Sumo deadlift Reverse lunge Cable pull through Standing Pallof press
Phase 2 (Specifics)	Front squat Single-leg hip thrust Glute hamstring raise Swiss-ball rollout	Barbell hip thrust Forward lunge Dumbbell RDL Running stance Pallof press
Phase 3 (Power)	Box jump Deadstop single-leg RDL Single-leg Swiss-ball leg curl Standing TRX rollout	Kettlebell swing High-box step-up Broad jump Kneeling Pallof press on both sides

But remember, weights and a gym membership, although helpful, aren't essential. You can build this strength at home using your bodyweight, too.

There's a principle called progressive overload that means you need to add weight or volume in order to get stronger. And so, with your bodyweight the load will be lighter, but you can increase the rep ranges to compensate.

However, as mentioned, with the addition of momentum, you have to be able to deal with forces greater than your bodyweight when running and so, at some point, you'll need some kind of external load to keep building strength. That doesn't have to be in a fancy gym; it can be with anything at home. A tin of paint from the shed? Hold it to your chest and squat. A two-litre bottle of water in each hand? Press them overhead. Get creative.

UPWARDLY MOBILE

Today, rightly so, there's been a trend towards mobility and activations before both runs and gym work. I'm a big fan, but with one major caveat: there's a big difference between mobility and flexibility and you shouldn't confuse the two.

Flexibility is your body's ability to move through a range of motion. Mobility is your body's ability to *actively* move through that range of motion. Let's think about yoga – yoga will allow you to get into some amazingly flexible positions *passively* because you're using the assistance of the floor, straps, or even the instructor who will help you to extend your range of movement. This is not to diss yoga, which is wonderful and makes people feel great, but this is not the active mobility that is so useful when you're looking to protect yourself against injury.

Active mobility is when you're able to access this level of flexibility yourself. Let me explain the difference. Take someone who has done plenty of yoga and stretching and is able to, when lying back on the floor, have somebody push their leg up and above their head. Now ask them to stand there and lift their leg up as high as they can. I'd bet they're only able to lift it out to hip height. That's the difference between an active range and a passive range.

The reason I mention this is because to injury-proof yourself the difference between active range and passive range needs to be as small as possible. And, perhaps confusingly, it's why a super-stiff, muscular front-row rugby player is probably better equipped to avoid injury than a bendy yogi. The reason is that, even though they might have a much smaller range of motion, they can access all of that range themselves, and they're strong as hell through all of it, too. They therefore can't get into a position where they're going to get injured. Any position they can get into, they own it and they're really strong.

On the other hand, your super-bendy person can get into all kinds of wacky positions, but they don't have any control there and can't activate their muscles at that end range. They can get there, they can relax and it can feel great, but if they're moving rather than being stationary on a mat they risk injury. That's because they can get into positions that they don't have the strength to get back from.

What this boils down to, therefore, is that flexibility for flexibility's sake is not a bonus athletically, because you can't use it. With mobility you can. And mobility starts with stability and using activations to build a connection between your brain and the muscle at its end range. That way you can then ensure all of your stretches are dynamic and involve getting into a position but then, crucially, having the stability to get back out again.

Stability starts by activating your core musculature, setting your abs tight and turning on your glutes. Turn everything on in the middle, and then with that control through your midsection and through your hips you can then start to build mobility as you get further out. So, when you work on your mobility, start at your core, glutes and hamstrings then move on to mobilise your hips, ankles, shoulders and thoracic spine.

With that in mind, this is the best way to build a simple mobility sequence that you can do before every workout:

The deadbug
You lay on your back with arms and legs up in the air and then lower alternately your opposite arm and leg. You're mimicking running with your arms and your legs while trying to maintain core activation by keeping your body stationary on the floor. That's the key: keeping your midsection and your

torso stable and braced while moving your limbs around that solid midsection.

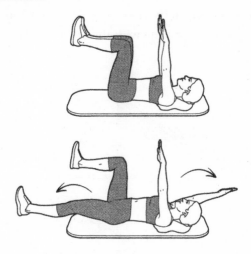

Glute bridges

Next comes glute bridges, which involve feet on the floor, driving your hips up to the air. This will switch on your glute muscles while keeping everything else braced, which is super important for runners.

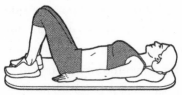

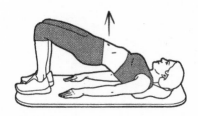

Dynamic pigeon

In a high plank position, you then lunge one leg forward and lay your glute and leg on the floor at 90 degrees before reversing the movement and repeating with the other leg. This takes care of your hips.

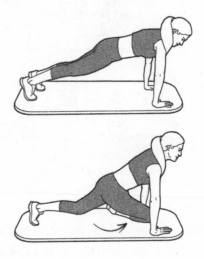

Side-lying windmills

Finally, for your shoulders and spine, the side-lying windmills are excellent. Lie on your side with your top leg, knee bent, resting on a foam roller. Then rotate your top arm from out in front of you, all the way around above your head, behind you, down below and back again before repeating on the opposite side.

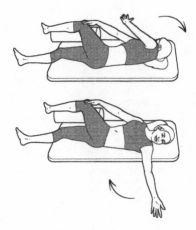

If you want to get really fancy you can sequence mobility exercises together which then starts to look a little bit like a little yoga flow, but fires up the body rather than chills it out.

Spend a few minutes doing this pattern below (repeating in the opposite direction) and you're primed to run and lift your way to a stronger, faster you.

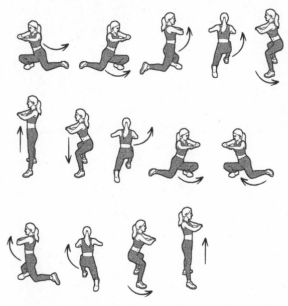

Your Chapter 5 Action Plan

- Stop running for every workout. You may be on a journey to become a runner, but there's more to it than mind-numbing mileage

- Remember: just as there's no one body shape for a runner, there's no one body shape for a lifter, either. Barbells do not equal bulk

- Familiarise yourself with the four main movement patterns and ensure any lifting plan contains plenty of them

- Get your deadlift technique on point! It's the one move to rule them all

- Start every workout, be that a run or barbell session, with a mobility flow

CHAPTER 6

The Art Of Doing F*ck All

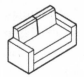

My Journey

As you read in the previous chapter, in order to become faster and fitter, and (as we've now established) lighter in my 20s, I assumed I needed to constantly do more. More midweek fasted exercise. More 7am gym sessions. More gruelling home HIIT. For a while, this worked. Both my body-fat percentage and mile times went in the right direction. Down. In treadmill classes, such as Barry's Bootcamp I channelled Dina Asher-Smith and, in shop changing rooms, I looked smugly in the mirror at my shrinking limbs and popping abs. My fitness life was going well until, of course, the day that it wasn't. And, it didn't just go from good to middling, it went from good to toxic. My seemingly healthy lifestyle was about to blow up in my face.

Despite breezily smashing out 50 burpees the day before, and sharing an egotistical Instagram about it, I found myself sitting in the corner of my living room crying uncontrollably with my arms wrapped around my knees. It's hard to describe the sense of fear I felt; all I wanted to do was run away from that room, run away from the immobilising sense of panic that appeared out of nowhere, took hold of my body and caused me to huddle by the side of the sofa. But I couldn't, I couldn't go anywhere. I felt too anxious to move. I'm not sure how long I spent with tears streaming down my cheeks and snot dripping on to my sports socks because in that moment, seconds felt like hours. When my flatmate finally walked into the room and repeatedly asked 'Who's been hurt?' thinking I was crying about bad news concerning a family member, I couldn't answer because the irony was, the person in pain was me.

RUNNING INTO DANGER

For the two years before, much like my healthy eating that started with good intentions, I'd gone from using exercise for self-improvement to a form of self-harm. As a health editor it's still shameful for me to admit that. But sadly, it's true. If I ate something 'bad', I ran. If I had a stressful day at work, I worked out. If I was tired, I sprinted the steps at the local football stadium for an 'energy boost'.

Scarcely a half hour of my day would go by when I didn't think about how and when I was going to exercise next – if I wasn't sticking my head down a toilet bowl to rid myself of the things I felt I needed to then I used compulsive exercise as a form of purging.

Exercise had become something I wouldn't go to bed without, which isn't uncommon for women suffering from eating disorders.

I remember one bitterly cold Christmas doing a workout in

my mum's garden wearing reindeer ears and gloves. At the time, I told myself it was healthy. Looking back on it, the healthier option would have been to not binge-eat the bowl of Lindt Lindor chocolates (the motivation to burpee) and instead have a cuppa and join in on the family movie.

But back then I didn't realise that exercise is a stress on the body and there's a tipping point beyond which the amount of exercise you perform can do more harm than good. Along with bulimia, the term overtraining syndrome (OTS) wasn't part of my vocabulary, nor was Relative Energy Deficiency in Sport (RED-S) – the consequences of which could compromise me mentally and physically, altering my metabolism, menstrual cycle, bone health, immunity and psychological health.

At the time I didn't give a second thought to how exercising hard and not eating enough – or purging – could impact my health. I lived for burning 500 calories and hitting the red zone in all workouts. However, my terrifying panic attack forced me to recognise that I'd ignored the warning signs (intermittent sleep, bad skin and no periods) and that I was exercising myself into the ground.

Unbeknown to me, constantly skipping rest and recovery, coupled with disordered eating, had caused internal warfare. Take my periods. My body felt under siege and had battened down the hatches to protect itself. There was no way it could preserve itself *plus* a baby so it skipped ovulation. To use medical speak, I was suffering from amenorrhea.

On the outside, the symptoms of something not being right were glaringly obvious for me to see. From my chin and spread across my jawline I had a constant run of acne. Big, sore cysts lived deep in the skin and were slow to heal. They scarred too. I spent my time and money trying to rid myself of them, eventually breaking down in a doctor's appointment and begging to be referred to a dermatologist to be put on Roaccutane – the controversial acne wonder drug. At no point though, did I pause to consider what was causing this hormonal acne, I just accepted the diagnosis and pushed on with treatment. Had I pressed the doctor for details I would have discovered that physical exercise can elevate cortisol, your body's stress hormone, and this is linked to increased oil production and a decreased ability to heal wounds. The combination can then manifest as problematic skin.

And it wasn't just the physical symptoms of overtraining and under-fuelling that I ignored. At work, I'd begun to suffer from unusual irritability and an inability to concentrate. My brain felt like Google Chrome with one too many tabs open and I regularly started my next task without finishing my last. My mind was chaotic and, more often than not, I was on the brink of losing my *shit* at my desk. To deal with it in the immediate term, I regularly shut out the world by closing my eyes to take big gulps of oxygen. My job was stressful – I managed the UK digital arm of a global brand – but I wasn't saving lives, so why did I constantly feel like I was in a state of emergency?

The relief came around three months after my panic attack. I'd felt a loss of energy and motivation to exercise so when offered the opportunity to train with a new PT – a perk of my health editor's role – I jumped at the chance. Of course, I started the session with demands of fat-burning exercises and questions alluding to weight loss, but unlike other personal-training experiences before, where PTs would simply acquiesce to my request, this was different. Luke Worthington (who you've just met) did not prescribe burpees or running up and down staircases in a weighted vest. Instead he chose to give it to me straight: 'You're chronically stressed,' he told me. 'Look at yourself right now, you're up on your toes, your ribs are flared and you look like you're about to have a fight.' He wasn't wrong. In that moment I wanted to fight the notion that something was wrong with me and knock him out in doing so. But I was also exhausted. And so, while debating whether the pile of exercise mats next to us would provide a comfy spot for a power nap, I conceded defeat and instead, allowed myself to be led through Luke's low-intensity session.

For the next 12 weeks I focused on nothing more than postural work, heavy weights and breathing patterns. No jump-jumpy workouts or intense training that drained my energy stores. I was beyond bored. I constantly questioned this training method's ability to deliver results because, deep down, I still yearned to be lighter and smaller. Then, my second meltdown of the year happened. I spent nearly 48 hours either sleeping or crying. There was no trigger to this depressive behaviour; I simply left work for the weekend and then physically and mentally collapsed.

On Monday I went back to the gym and retold my woeful weekend to Luke who simply smiled (the second time I wanted to lamp him in almost as many months) and replied: 'That's what happens when your highly strung nervous system finally gets a rest.'

SYSTEM FAILURE

The body is a highly intelligent thing. At times, it can also be rather dumb. Actually, that's not fair. Not dumb, but not in tune with modern life. For instance, let's talk about the 'fight-or-flight' response. As humans have evolved we've gained internal wiring that acts as a survival mechanism, reacting immediately when there's a risk of danger. Millennia ago, said danger was escaping the gnarly teeth of sabre-tooth tigers and other predators out for a pound of flesh. Today, the danger is different but our body reacts in the same way as it did in prehistory. A looming work deadline, bitchy WhatsApp exchange or 200m of hill sprints are processed in the same way as that tiger on our tails. And, therein lies the problem.

Unlike years ago when stressful situations would come and go, in today's world, stress surrounds us. There is little opportunity to switch off the stress hormones coursing through our bodies.

Stress, when experienced in short bursts, isn't bad. However, when experienced chronically it can take its toll on physical and psychological health. This is what happened to me. Exposing my body to constant stress – through work and workouts – forced my body to continually stimulate the sympathetic nervous system (the one responsible for getting me out of danger). And at no point did I take my foot off the gas and allow my parasympathetic nervous system (responsible for 'rest and digest') to kick in.

Not only that, I worked out to torch cals and burn fat. However, the workouts were only adding to my stress, further elevating cortisol. All of which combined to curtail any chance I had of actually achieving those goals. A cursory glance at the Harvard Health website made clear that too much cortisol can contribute to the buildup of fat tissue, increased appetite and weight gain. Which is pretty fucking stressful. Without realising it, I'd become locked into a never-ending stress cycle.

NEW FOUNDATIONS

To put the brakes on my skyrocketing stress levels, Worthington had put the brakes on my workouts. I took an enforced breather on breathless sessions and under no circumstances was I to train twice a day, or more than four times a week. From then on each workout session began with deep abdominal breathing and the rest periods between each exercise were longer than work periods (a rare occurrence in mainstream HIIT or tread-mill sprint sessions). I rebooted and recalibrated my relationship with exercise for the better.

Fast-forward to today and I'm now aware that my exercise life and normal life are not mutually exclusive. They are more entwined than the cast of *Love Island*. It's why these days you won't find me fighting a stressful day with a stressful workout, nor will you find me chasing a Sunday long run with a Monday-morning HIIT session. Instead, I train mindfully, not more, to minimise the impact of cardio on my cortisol. As a result I'm stronger, faster, more energised, clear-headed and happier than before. I haven't had a spot in weeks, either.

Taking steps to improve your health and fitness is undeniably laudable, but there's a limit. If you can feel yourself chasing after too much of a good thing, it's time you gave yourself a break.

'If you feel
tired learn to
rest, not quit'

Follow The Leader

Researchers at the St. Vincent Sports Performance Center believe that a large percentage of the people who train for 10ks, half marathons and marathons are overtrained by the time they reach the starting line.[25] *A very high percentage get into a state of fatigue that they just cannot get out of. Joslyn Thompson Rule wants to change that. She is a strength coach and Nike Master Trainer in London who is passionate about training smarter not harder. Her advice will help you to achieve better progress from a process that is more enjoyable and able to safeguard both your mental and physical health. Join her in the slow lane.*

It seems strange to start worrying about people doing *too much* exercise, when so many people struggle to lace up their trainers in the first place. But it has increasingly become an issue, and one that is sabotaging your ability to make progress – and if left unchecked, may start to impact your health.

LOOK OUT FOR RED FLAGS

These symptoms hint that you're overtraining:

- A general level of fatigue. It's a feeling of exhaustion that you just can't seem to shake, even when you think you're doing a lot of things right and healthily in your day-to-day.

- Lack of motivation. This could even develop further and be described as a low level of depression.

- Little niggles that won't go away.

- General underperformance in your actual training,

when you're just not able to hit what should be target weights, times and paces in a session.

- Insomnia. Difficulty getting to sleep or staying asleep can be an indication of overtraining, or under recovery.

HIT THE RESET BUTTON

If you recognise any of these symptoms then a rest day will no longer cut it. You've gone too far and your body needs to properly power down. My prescription would be a week off training, in the gym or on the road, and limiting yourself to three walks throughout the week. Getting outside and into nature will be crucial in allowing you to reverse what's happening in your body and bring your stress levels down.

Another benefit of walking is that it's an excuse to get off your phone (leave it at home!). This forces you to slow down physically and mentally. It's also amazing what you can work through in your head without distraction – using that time to clear through your mental to-do list will leave you with a noticeable sense of calm when you return home. I won't say it's easy, because I think it's hard for people who are in that always-on cycle to break it, but walking is a really good start.

After doing that for a week, reintroduce everything at 50 per cent effort. Do half the miles and lift half the weights for half the reps. Then add another 10 per cent the next week, and another 10 per cent the next. All the while, have in the back of your head a constant checking for an approaching tipping point. It may be frustrating to be operating at half speed, but it's necessary, and if you're smart about it then the comeback process will provide a useful framework to work out how far you can push yourself so that you never risk overdoing it again.

The best part will come when you reach a point of training at the correct intensity. After weeks of redlining, followed by weeks of recovery and getting back up to speed, the progress you'll be able to make when you strike the correct balance between training and rest will be worth the wait.

The best example of this is the office worker who trains five days a week, eats OK, but has a stressful job, and their progress has plateaued. No matter how many HIIT classes or tempo runs they do, they don't seem to be getting any faster or leaner. Then, when they go away on holiday, after doing hardly any training, eating what they want and having a few drinks – they actually end up losing weight. That's all because they're more relaxed. Despite the contradiction of doing less and eating more, their body is in a chilled-out state where it can do what it bloody well needs to.

IT STARTS IN THE MIND

More useful than an action plan to reset after overtraining (or under-recovery, my preferred term) are pointers to stop you from reaching that point in the first place. And I've alluded to it already, but the mental stresses of life can play an equal, if not greater, part in causing burnout than the physical stresses of training.

You want to look at it holistically. There's only a certain amount of stress that the body can take and this is split between the physical and mental. This becomes problematic when people all too often attempt to cure their mental anxieties with physical exertion.

If you can imagine a glass, and you fill it up nearly to the brim, and think of that as the mental stress of work and home life. Then you add exercise to that – even if it's something super-simple – it will overflow and that signifies the breakdown of overtraining or under-recovery. There's a really fine balance of how much exercise is enough to reduce mental stress. In the short term it releases endorphins and you can enjoy the high that you get post-exercise. Long term, however, chasing this high with increasingly hard workouts can become a really, really big problem.

Unfortunately, when people are highly stressed they will often choose to go to something like a boxing class – which is high intensity – to punch away the stresses of the day, and it doesn't work. That's because they may already be taxing their system with office meetings and childcare.

The after-class high is so short-lived, but it's also all that you remember. And so you chase it. A perfect example is one woman who used to come to a HIIT class I taught, and I recognised that she was coming all the time. Before I could step in, though, at the end of one session she burst into tears in the changing room. She basically had a breakdown; she was feeling down and not feeling motivated. I explained to her that she was simply doing too much training. She was chasing a high that she never reached and her obvious response was to do more in the hope she would eventually get there.

It's very hard to tell somebody to slow down, especially alpha types who are in the middle of a big city, competing because they need to get ahead in life, let alone in the gym. But recognising and being mindful of where you're at and what you're dealing with outside of your training plan will help to keep you moving forward in a positive way.

MAKE TIME TO CHECK IN

As a coach it is my responsibility to be able to see when my client is overtrained. And that's why you may notice a PT asking you the same innocuous questions every time you come in the gym. How are you feeling? How did you sleep? I'll also be looking at how you walk into the gym and how you're sitting – anything that can help to gauge where you're at physically and mentally. But you don't need a PT to benefit, you can track yourself.

I think, generally speaking, the more you track, the more empowered you are to make decisions about your own health. But that comes with a small caveat in that if you get too obsessed then it can morph into something negative. It's a fine line.

My issue with tech, while it's wonderful on one hand, is that it can disassociate us from what our bodies are telling us. I really don't trust when that relationship of 'how am I feeling in this moment' is handed over to technology. And the problem then also becomes paralysis by over-analysis. The level of detail on devices can leave you stumped as to where to start. The best way is to simplify the analytical stuff and give yourself a rating out of 10. Ask yourself the following:

- How hard was your training session?
- How well have you eaten on any given day overall – did you eat enough, and was there a mix of protein, carbohydrates and fat?
- Did you drink enough water?
- How stressed are you at work?
- How did you sleep?

Give yourself a mark out of 10 for each throughout the week. If you're feeling low, lack motivation or feel like your training has slowed down come Sunday, then these scores will give you an indication of where you need to focus your attentions or take your foot off the pedal.

COMPARING WORKOUTS

If you find it tough to work out the relative physical and mental toll of your training sessions, this scoring system from running coach Anthony Fletcher will help. Multiply the rate of perceived exertion (score how tough you found it out of 10) by the number of minutes you were exercising.

Compare a HIIT session that takes 30 minutes, exercising at 9/10 with a Sunday long run for 60 minutes at 4/10, for example.

HIIT: $30 \times 9 = 270$

Long run: $60 \times 4 = 240$

Despite being half the duration, the HIIT session actually took a higher toll on your body and requires more time to recover from. Consider this when you extend that HIIT session to the 60 minutes of the standard workout class and you can see why they're a shortcut to overtraining if you're not careful . . .

START THE RECOVERY PROCESS

Keeping tabs on your training intensity and your nutrition are key points in ensuring you're well recovered. But there are more ways you can maximise that process. Here I run the rule over some of the different ways to make more of your down time.

Active recovery

This may be a buzz phrase, but it's an important tool that gives pride of place to the practice of going *slow*. When you're tired, gentle movement to induce blood flow will aid in recovery. For some people that's walking or swimming, for others it might be a lighter session in the gym, like some gentle sled-pushing. It can be anything that creates some kind of movement through your body to activate blood flow.

Stretching

You can just do some good old stretching. I'm old-fashioned in this case and simply taking 5, 10 or 15 minutes to move your body through some stretches or mobility work can work wonders. Although you can't truly change the length of muscles, in addition to improving blood flow, stretching can encourage better range and fluid movement through your joints, which will aid recovery.

Depending on the style, yoga can be active. For recovery you want a more zen type of yoga, rather than a dynamic yoga – but again that depends on your fitness. If you're fitter and stronger you would be less affected by a dynamic yoga session.

Massage

What this does, again, is to increase blood flow. It helps to get blood into the muscles and into the tissues. This influx of oxygen and removal of lactic acid helps to speed up the recovery process. And there's the relaxation effect, obviously. The right massage can provide a moment to recover mentally as well as physically. And, as you now know, giving yourself some head space can increase your ability to train and progress physically. It depends on the masseuse, though! Not all massages are that comfortable . . .

With foam-rolling, people are up in the air about that because it doesn't loosen muscles, it's more of a neurological effect. It's understood there may be some benefits from foam-rolling after a session to aid recovery, but research is still in its infancy.

Recovery tools

If you've scrolled through your Instagram feed you've likely come face-to-face with a percussive massage gun, or recovery gun to use it's other name. You know, the ones that look like a power drill but position themselves to help with everything from muscle stress, pain and tissue tension to enhanced recovery, blood circulation and range of motion. If you decide to use one of these handheld massage tools be aware that although these tools may leave you with the immediate sense of feeling great, by design, they do hammer down on muscle tissue. Pummelling away may not mean that your muscles are actually *recovering*, they may just feel better, which could put you at risk of falling into a false sense of security and training too hard too soon.

Sleep

Sleep is when your body adapts to all of the hard work that you're putting in. The change doesn't happen when you're in the gym, the adaptation to exercise happens when you're at rest. If you're not getting enough rest that adaptation can't occur. It's absolutely crucial.

To improve yours, cut back on caffeine throughout the day and introduce a cut-off point at 2pm. Go analogue in the evening and read a book in bed instead of scrolling your phone. And, much like the theme for this section, slow down!

Hot or cold?

And finally, cryotherapy or saunas? Hot shower or cold bath? There are plenty of options at either end of the spectrum that purport to benefit your recovery from exercise. And many of you will be pleased to learn that the emerging research suggests that heat has the edge.

Yes, the Wim Hof method is trending and cold-water swimming is now seen as a health panacea, but in terms of recovery the most exciting area of research is edging towards saunas. Far from being the easy way out of slacking in the gym, combining time in the sauna with an effective week of workouts can help you to recover more quickly and make more progress as you do. Consider that my final hot tip.

THE INS AND OUTS OF HRV

With Simon Wegerif of Myithlete

HRV stands for heart-rate variability. It's different from the heart-rate measurement that you would get first thing in the morning or while you're out training. Instead, it measures the precise time gaps between heartbeats as you breathe in and when you breathe out. These tiny differences are able to tell you about the body's nervous and regulatory control systems,

---

which are useful in helping you to decide how stressed or recovered you are.

Most people think that while you're sitting at rest that your heart is beating like a metronome. For example, if you have a resting heart rate of 60 beats per minute, that means there's a beat every second. Well, that's not the case. There is variation, and the way that that changes can tell you a lot about your body's readiness to perform.

The ideal is lots of variability, particularly between when you breathe in and when you breathe out. As you breathe in your heart should accelerate and when you breathe out your heart goes more slowly. It's the reason that when you take a deep breath during your yoga flow or meditation you instantly feel calmer.

As the heart slows down you become more parasym-pathetic dominant and the parasympathetic nervous system is the part that's responsible for rest, digestion and recovery. And it's that part that we want to be able to measure every day to tell if your body has been able to recover properly and whether you're in any danger of overtraining when you're preparing for a marathon.

How to take your HRV

To measure HRV you'll need a heart-rate sensor and an app that processes the data, like ithlete. After waking each morning, relax and sit comfortably, slip on a chest strap or finger sensor and follow the on-screen instructions to get an accurate reading of your HRV.

Low HRV

The lower the HRV the more stressed your body is. In fact, a constant heart rate is the sign of a very, very stressed body. Think of it like you're stretching an elastic band out to as far as it can go. It's incredibly tense and there's little to no movement.

High HRV

This implies that your body is very capable of adapting to its environment and performing at its best.

Normal HRV

In truth, there is no one 'normal' HRV as it's what's normal for you. Your HRV fluctuates greatly throughout the day, from one day to the next, and generally decreases with age. What's better than asking 'what should my HRV be?' is to ask, 'What is a good HRV trend for me?'

HRV trends

Training is all about stress and recovery, so the aim should be to take a reading of your HRV every morning. The more readings you compile, the better you can determine what your baseline reading is.

A hard session will lower your HRV number, while a rest day of recovery should increase your HRV. If your HRV stays low even with rest, you could be moving towards trouble. That's why you want to be aware of your baseline number and how this is affected by your day-to-day and training.

Factors that play with your HRV

The factors that affect your HRV can be split into three categories: training, lifestyle and biological.

Training factors:

- New workouts
- Volume of work
- Intensity of workouts
- Frequency of workouts

Lifestyle factors:

- Nutrition
- Alcohol
- Stress
- Sleep

Biological factors:

- Age
- Gender
- Genetics
- Health conditions

THE STRESS TEST FOR RUNNERS

If your HRV is higher than baseline in the morning then all is well; you're fully recovered and ready to train as hard as you like, be that through intervals or a tempo session. However, if your HRV is lower than normal then it's a sign that you're not fully recovered. This doesn't mean you need to stop everything and step away from the treadmill but you might want to modify your session to lessen the duration or intensity; choose a slightly less intense or slightly shorter workout on that day. If your HRV is significantly below your baseline, particularly for two days in a row, then you need to take that as a sign that the body is stressed and it needs more time to recover before you're ready to go out again.

It's been shown that the risk of soft-tissue injuries and illness is greatly increased when people train all-out on days where they're tracking low HRV. And it's easily done, especially when training for a marathon and the body is being forced into making a major step up from Parkruns. The injury statistics are not good. Around 30 per cent of runners will have their marathon training plans disrupted by injury or sickness. HRV, although in its infancy, provides another simple measure that you can do every morning when you wake up to help you to make healthy, long-term progress.

On The Run With . . . Natalie Lawrence

We live in an era where punishing workouts are celebrated in the gym and validated on social media. But when it comes to exercise, you really can have too much of a good thing. There are many triggers that can push a noble pursuit of fitness to become a negative, but for Natalie Lawrence, a semi-pro triath-lete and personal trainer, it was misplaced advice from her coaches that triggered an obsession with fitness. Within months she was waking at 5am to swim 6k, then doing two three-hour sessions of running or cycling and gym work every day. She cut out all carbohydrates, employed a 'half' rule where she would eat only half the meal on her plate, and occasionally suffered from bulimia. Today she is well on the road to recovery. On our run together, the mother of four explains how she has recalibrated her priorities and, through her work as a personal trainer, come to appreciate exercise for the joy that's in it.

AL: Has training always been a part of your life? Did the motivation to exercise begin as a kid?

NL: I've always done it. Both my sister and I channelled our childhood energies into running and we moved up through county and national levels until about 16.

From there I moved on to biathlon, which is a run and a swim. At the nationals I'd been seeded second and came second, and I ended up being talent scouted to move into a funded programme for British triathlon. I then continued trialling and went to the Junior World Champs and the Europeans. I eventually went off to university to study, but also became part of the high-performance group where I could live and train with the squad.

AL: That's all very high pressure and all-consuming from a very young age. Did you have time for any other interests as a kid or teenager?

NL: Nothing really. Excuse the pun, but I always say to people now that I jumped into the deep end. I was put on funding and in my first ever triathlon I was trying to qualify to get into the Great Britain youth team. I didn't do it just to finish the race. I didn't do it as a novice. I had to do it in a high-pressure situation. And obviously, I did crap. I panicked. I didn't know about transitions.

If I reflect on it today I feel robbed of doing it and loving it. I've never loved triathlons. If anything, I'm only starting to learn to love it now, because now I'm the only one putting on pressure. But from my teenage years upwards I've only ever known training, swimming, discipline, minimal social time and not really deviating into any other sport or leisure activity.

AL: When a lot of people don't want to do exercise, they just don't do it. But you weren't in that kind of environment. If you were having to grind out training sessions and you didn't want to be there, what was going through your head at that time?

NL: I was driven personally, but I admit there was a little bit of pressure at home to deal with. I always maintain, though, that if I ever wanted to stop, especially as I got older, I could have done. I said the minute I was doing it for someone else, I wouldn't do it.

AL: Was it the success that was addictive? What was it that maintained your drive?

NL: I think I saw potential in myself. Obviously being put on funding and being scouted made me think, 'Well I must be doing something right.' In many ways I did enjoy the process. I became used to the drills and the training. Really, though, it was the competing that I enjoyed and the carrot dangling in front of me – the chance of making the GB team.

AL: At what time did your relationships with exercise and food change?

NL: Pretty much the first time we were training with the squad as freshers, the girls and boys were taken to the weights room where we did strength and conditioning and we were weighed. At that time I didn't even know what kilograms were and what they meant to me.

AL: So you'd never weighed yourself before that point?

NL: Never. I'd never needed to. I just used my body as a tool and I didn't think I was particularly small, but also I didn't think I was big, and I was doing all right. But then performance became the drive and I spent time with nutritionists who explained I could lean up, slim down and get a bit quicker. It made sense. You're carrying your bodyweight in running, so you're expending more energy the more weight you're carrying.

AL: That's a very complex issue to start messing with! What was your diet like before that?

NL: It could have been better if I'm honest. But you've got to remember at the time I was living at home, and I didn't always have the luxury of cooking my own meals, and I certainly didn't buy and bring in my own food. My mum knew that once we got in from swim training – that's a 2–2½ hour training session – we would just smash through a load of food and pretty much go straight to bed. Even my friends back in the day would say the food portions I was able to put away were amazing.

AL: But you were burning through hundreds and hundreds of calories . . .

NL: Exactly. We were in the water at 5am for 2 hours, school, and then 2 hours in the evening.

AL: That must have been a difficult thing to be confronted with by the coaches, then? If you've gone from feeling that food was fuel and you could smash through epic portions after long sessions, but were then being told that actually no, you still need to watch what you ate and should aim to lose weight, not just get faster – that can't have been easy?

NL: I went into it naïvely and I don't think we got full support from the nutritionists. It was very generic advice: we were all different heights and weights, we were all doing different training blocks, but it was a one-size-fits-all approach to food. We weren't all going to lose the same amount of weight with that plan.

At that time, I was watching the wrong things online, shadowing the wrong people and so my focus became more on my body, and less on what I was actually training and doing.

AL: Did that conversation about your weight change your eating ethos from fuelling performance to achieving a size that you believed would make you go faster, then?

NL: Yeah. And that's made more hardcore by the cut-throat nature of the environment. You get to that point you need results fast because that's the industry. They can't wait for you.

AL: How did your relationship with exercise begin to deteriorate? It had always been a competitive thing, but when was it that you noticed there was something changing and that it was no longer having a positive effect?

NL: It's a control thing. It is all-consuming. It's self-competitive. I definitely think there is a certain personality, which I am, that makes you more susceptible to these disorders. And that is something you need to be aware of and look out for in yourself. I now have friends who say, 'I want to achieve this this and this,' but in the next sentence they've said, 'Do you know what, I'll just have a Domino's.' And I can't relate to that because I think if I'm going to focus on something, I'm going to go and do it. And that's what happened between me and training.

I was in a high-pressure squad situation and there was competition between us. It became, 'Right, I'm going to do an extra session just to be one up on them.' I believed it would make me thinner, it would make me fitter. Then lines between a training plan that is designed to help me develop and just doing more and more exercise in the hope it'll make me quicker became blurred. It gets too much, your body breaks down and, coupled with poor nutrition, my body just gave up.

AL: And this is so important: making sure that people know that more is not always better. Thankfully recovery is something that people are talking about more and more, like eating well, resting and getting enough sleep. It's those things that can help you to go faster. How long were you stuck in this destructive relationship with training?

NL: Pretty much my whole time at university. I was meant to do three years but due to suffering from an eating disorder I had to extend it to four years. By that fourth period I had been demoted from the squad and had my funding cut because I just wasn't hitting the results. But there were obvious reasons for that.

The coaches dealt with it really badly. I ended up doing my dissertation on dealing with bulimia, and wrote about my time there without naming anyone, then sent it to the coaches. They did read it and held a meeting with me and apologised for how badly they had coped with it. I also got them to say that, with female athletes in particular, they'd take better care with things in the future.

AL: Did your relationship with exercise recover quickly when the pressure of competition was lifted, or was this new association between exercise and weight equally harmful?

NL: It was still a self-destruct thing. It was habitual, and I just carried on. A little bit of me had the hope that I could get back on the squad and bounce back, but it wasn't going to happen.

AL: Was there a turning point when it came to your relationship with exercise? From being focused on yourself as an athlete to then wanting to help and advise others as a trainer yourself – that surely requires a different mindset?

NL: That was it. It was nice for me to train and coach people who were doing it to start with, who hadn't had the journey that I had and who were literally just trying to get around a race. That was really quite inspiring to see. For me it was a final realisation that you can do all this without aspiring to be a certain level, or a certain weight.

If you look at the pyramid of it, mass participation is absolutely huge compared to where I was near the top. There's a lot fewer people in that catchment. It has been nice for me to rub shoulders with an attitude that I should have adopted from the beginning.

I don't know, it's hard. I would almost say that I was learning to love it how they love it. Because it was a different type of enjoyment to how I view it.

AL: How do you treat rest and recovery now?

NL: I still don't like going through a day when I'm not training. I still have the voice, very small in the back of my head saying, 'You don't really need a rest day, you don't even train that hard or that much any more to qualify for it.' But then on other days with four kids who are five and under, they're a training session in themselves; that coupled with a few workout classes is demanding both physically and mentally so I have to take a rest.

AL: I've only recently been learning the impact that mental stress has on top of physical stress. And on top of that just what a major part sleep plays in being able to recover and help to support healthy training habits. That can be hard to come by when you're a new parent, I imagine?!

NL: Yeah, I've had to work for it, but I've made sleep a priority. Even when all four of them are home at the weekend, I'm drilled now to get them upstairs for a nap around 1:30, which gives me a window of two hours and I actually use that time to sleep myself.

AL: Do you still find yourself struggling to deal with empty time and missed sessions?

NL: Yes, it's hard. Even when I've got two of them still asleep upstairs and two being picked up from school, I'm in a bit of no-man's-land. I think, Argh, I could have gone and done a session, I've got this time before I have to go out and work. But I've got children now. We always reflect, my husband and I, about all the time we had pre-kids! But that's why whenever I get a window of opportunity, I take it to train. They're only short, though – I make them quality. There are no junk miles.

AL: That's an encouraging shift from 'more is more' to doing it right . . . And you're back competing from time to time, too. What are you doing at the moment? How does your relationship with exercise exist now?

NL: I did the half Iron Man down in Weymouth. It was me winging it, and then unbeknown to me I got second in my age group and qualified for the Worlds! So next, it's the world champs in New Zealand! Again, it was like, 'Oh god, what could I do if I actually trained for it?'

AL: That's incredible! Maybe that's just further proof of how well you can do when your body is well rested. To go and compete in events now – are you able to exercise now for the enjoyment?

NL: Yeah, I do. It's nice to go out without a training plan to stick to. If I feel like pushing it, then I do. If I don't, no worries, I've got no real game plan. I do have hopes of introducing a bit more structure but I'm careful now, and aware that it's not ever going to reach the point where it takes over my life or pushes out the enjoyment. It's about finding a balance between a sense of accomplishment and also having fun.

AL: As a PT, but also talking directly to people who may well see themselves in your story, what advice would you give? How do you now view the importance of rest and recovery?

NL: When you're not enjoying what you're doing that's when you need to recognise a red flag and analyse why you're doing something. You can forget the how and the when, you just need to work out the why. If you're entering a race and your aim is to finish, then take the pressure off – you just need to get round without injury. If you want more, then you'll need more structured training, and that's OK. But the key then is to make sure that what you want is attainable in the timeframe that you have. When you put yourself under time pressure, I think that's when you start to beat yourself up and overdo it. The process should be enjoyable, not just the end result. If you put the training in and look after your body, the results will come.

Your Chapter 6 Action Plan

- Recognise that more isn't always better when it comes to training

- Dial back your workouts when work and life stresses build up, to protect yourself against burning out

- Listen to your body and regularly check in with how you're feeling using a score out of 10

- From the sauna to HRV tracking, experiment with different ways to help the recovery process. And prioritise sleep!

- Focus on your why. Decide on what is driving your workouts and make sure enjoyment takes pride of place

---

CHAPTER 7

Let's Call It A Comeback

My Journey

No running journey is straightforward. And it certainly isn't painless. But with a little extra knowledge, and a whole lot more self-care, I've gone from soothing shin splints with wine coolers to a winning attitude that now affords my mental and physical well-being pride of place.

Nothing sinks your enthusiasm for exercise quite so fast as an injury. Believe me, I know. When it happened, it wasn't the searing pain up the sides of my shins that bothered me (although it was bloody excruciating!) it was the mental sting of opportunity lost and progress wasted that was so tough to accept.

The way I acted was like a teenager who'd been told their boyfriend wasn't allowed to spend the night. I huffed. I became instantly frustrated: all the weeks I'd spent going to bed early with a box-set so that I could wake up fresh and ready to run before work now seemed pointless. And I was certain that without running I was going to gain weight and my fitness levels would plummet. Getting injured wasn't just physical pain, it was mental torture.

Importantly, that frustration distracted me from the fact that, well, it was my fault. It was *my* fault that I was sitting in the living room with frozen wine coolers around my legs because I'd ignored the early warning signs and trained through the pain. Although I look back and admire my grit and all-in attitude, my inexperience meant that I'd exercised through discomfort and was on the road to a stress fracture. I'd been foolhardy, and it ended up scuppering my plans to run three half marathons in three weeks and get consistently faster.

Although the half marathon challenge that I'd set myself didn't mean anything to anyone else, at the time it was my sole focus. Exercise had become my social life and it filled time that otherwise would have been spent on the sofa in my disgusting flat-share with its discoloured carpets.

And so, for three months, I ran and ran and ran. Until one day, I couldn't. I was injured and it broke me. As I sat on my sofa it felt like my access card to a world unburdened by life's pressures had been deactivated.

But dealing with injury is something everyone has to manage, no matter what level they're at. For example, twenty-something me was experiencing just a tiny serving of what Serena Williams went through at the start of her career – and just look where she is now. In 2006, Williams entered the Australian Open. She played, and subsequently lost to, Daniela Hantuchová. A knee injury was offered up as one of the reasons why. However, when Williams' biography hit bookshelves it became clear that this was only part of the story. Unbeknown to the thousands of spectators in Melbourne's stadium, Williams was also suffering from depression, and the subsequent layoff from injury served to exacerbate her ill-health.

Since that summer, Williams has rebuilt herself physically and mentally many times, all under the microscope of the media. She's become a spokesperson for psychological distress, especially after giving birth, and has continually proved that serious injury doesn't have to mean the end. Not all comebacks have the romance of high-profile sports, but that doesn't make your or my recovery from shin splints to complete a maiden half marathon any less inspiring or insightful. Because before you think it's only you that's been scuppered by the mundane, while others are brought down in a blaze of glory, think again.

Recently, the running gods answered my prayers and I was given the opportunity to run with Dame Kelly Holmes, who told me that before winning double gold she too suffered from injury. Hers was caused simply by swapping her running trainers to a style that weren't right for her pronation. She ran through pain, thinking it was merely an adjustment period, but ended up developing a bone stress injury and missing out on the medal she was so desperate for. It would be another eight years before Holmes collected gold in the 800m and 1500m to become a double Olympic champion. And then there's my bridesmaid who, eager to lose weight for my wedding decided to increase her mileage from zero to 15 miles in a week. She ran the same the week after. By week three she couldn't jog let alone run because her knees had swollen so badly. An MRI revealed she'd torn her anterior cruciate ligaments (ACL) and was given a rehabilitation time of six to nine months.

It's clear that knowing when to push on and when to pull back is a skill that even the greatest athletes get wrong. Injury, no matter how big or small, can be a physical and emotional drain. But it doesn't have to be the end. Since my agonising suspected stress fracture (not forgetting the hours of self-care wrapping wine coolers around my shins) I've gone on to run two marathons and a triathlon. Holmes got her gold and Williams, well, she's a global sporting icon. So, if your running pains have caused you to faceplant a bag of Maltesers in the recent past – not to mention consider a switch to the more leisurely hobby of lawn bowls – don't. With the right advice you can learn how to bulletproof your body and injury-proof your running to ensure your cardio career is defined by success, not setbacks.

'I'm down but I'm not out'

Follow The Leader

Brad Scanes is a specialist musculoskeletal physiotherapist who works with British gymnastics teams. He specialises in helping his regular clients to prevent and overcome running injuries. Here he is to share his expertise. Listen up . . .

SORE KNEES

It'll come as little surprise that the most common running injury is knee pain. There are various types, but the most common is patellofemoral syndrome. Which sounds pretty horrendous, I admit! However, it's simply an umbrella term of scientific jargon. The patellofemoral joint is that between the kneecap and the femur (your thigh bone) and there are plenty of structures behind the kneecap that can become inflamed during running. And that's where the pain comes from – you know the one, the one you can't really put your finger on. It feels internal and deep and, well, that's because it is. It's happening in the tissue behind your kneecap.

As with a lot of running injuries it's the result of repetitive stress. That's fancy talk for overuse. In fact, 80 per cent of injuries are to do with training error and that invariably is down to overeager runners trying to do too much too soon. Newbies will go from 5k to 8k to 10k in a matter of weeks, if not days. They're ignoring one of the golden rules for runners: you should only ever increase your mileage by 10 per cent from week to week. Follow this simple format and you will easily lower your risk of repetitive-stress injuries.

But remember, it's best to think about the 10 per cent rule over the course of a week, rather than on individual runs – otherwise it gets too complicated too quickly. Record how much you did the week before in mileage or minutes and then work out how far to push on the following week. If you ran 20 miles over four runs, then the next week you could run 22 over five shorter runs or three longer runs. It allows you to have some leeway to work your training around your schedule with a little common sense. Which means cramming it all into one 22-mile run is out of the question, obviously.

If you're a beginner determined for faster progression there is some evidence that, in the lower distances, you can probably extend that mileage increase to 15 or 20 per cent. If you're already up and running big mileage each week, then you're safer sticking to 10 per cent.

The second way you can prevent this kind of injury centres on the issue of capacity. When you're running, the force exerted on your knees is somewhere between four and seven times your bodyweight. That's a lot for one joint to take and so you need to call in reinforcements. The simplest way to do this is with strength and conditioning in the gym, which you should know from chapter 5. By building up your quadricep muscles, glutes, hamstrings and calves, these strong muscle tissues can act as shock absorbers for your joints and protect you from pain.

A lot of people during their training are forced to do it on pavements, which is by far the most unforgiving surface on your joints. The way to minimise this, beyond adding leg strength, is to look at your shoes. Choosing a different shoe altogether isn't always the problem, but more often than not it's needing to update the shoe you're running in. There's a lot of different research but I would suggest investing in an update of your runners every 300–500 miles on the road.

SHIN SPLINTS

Shin splints, by definition, are an exertional pain on the inside border of the shin bone. Once again, it has a scary umbrella term – medial tibial stress syndrome, but this can relate to 30 different pathologies. It's on the spectrum of bone-stress injuries. At one end you have a stress fracture, which is *serious* and why running through shin pain is never a smart idea. At the other end of the continuum you have the more benign dysfunctions in the muscles and tendons surrounding the shin bone, plus the potential for pain in the lining of the bone itself. In most cases it is a combination of all these things. In short, it's complicated! Which is why, sadly, there's not a simple fix.

To remedy the situation you need to work out why this has come on. The best way to do it is to review a snapshot of the previous four weeks' training. If you've unwittingly added more than 30 per cent mileage compared to last week then your risk of injury all of a sudden skyrockets by four times.

I never like to stop people from running, but because of the continuum shin splints sit on (alongside stress fractures) sometimes that's the only option; you need to be mindful of the risks. But there's also an element of playing it by ear, too, and listening to your body. If you're OK to walk and run a little bit, then that's fine. If you can run for 5k pain-free, but then pain sets in at 6k, then that's something to bear in mind. 5k is your starting point. You can keep running and you can cross-train the rest of your training to ensure you don't lose fitness while the inflammation settles down.

Types of cross-training for runners
- Cycling
- Swimming

- Aqua jogging
- Elliptical machine
- SkiErg machine

In addition to these cross-training techniques, you can use other techniques like icing and elevation to speed up that process.

There are other accessories that you can look into while you're not running, to ensure you can be pain-free more quickly. You need to increase load tolerance. I get my clients to do a lot of hopping particularly multi-directional hopping to increase the robustness of their bone and tissue. Equally, the calf is actually the most important muscle for runners; not only will it protect against injury, but there's a lot of research to say that the stronger it is the faster you'll go. But more on that later.

PLANTAR FASCIITIS

This condition, which we now call plantar fasciopathy, is a degenerative problem that affects the fascia – a thick band of tissue on the bottom of your foot. As with all these injuries, it sounds worse than it is. All that degenerative means is that the tissue itself is breaking down a little.

Fascia, like a tendon, is involved in transferring load. It has a certain capacity, but if it is continually pushed beyond that capacity without the adequate recovery then the tissue breaks down and becomes sore. Simple, really.

But there is an important differentiation to make, because rest will take away the pain but that pain will immediately reappear once you get back to running. If the tissue is broken down, rest won't build it back. You need to add strength work and rehabilitation to recover and build up its capacity for pounding pavements *ad nauseam*.

So, yes, you should stop running if you keep feeling the pain. But, as with the other injuries, it's about working out what you can do pain-free and using that as the start point for your rehab. Early intervention does speed up recovery – and I'm not just saying that because I want more clients!

People are guilty of ignoring all sorts of things, whether that's at the doctor or the dentist; however, to make this specific to running, when you've been in pain for a while you experience physical changes. Pain forces your body to find a new way to do the same movement or makes you stop doing it altogether. You lose muscle mass, and if your strength is reducing then you'll exacerbate the problem of moving in different ways. Other muscles will kick in to compensate and a domino effect of injuries to these newly-relied-upon muscles will occur. It's a two-for-one deal you really, really don't want.

The best rehab I've found for this is relatively simple. It's a version of the calf raise where you place a folded towel under your big toe and do the exercise with the toe slightly elevated. This will target the fascia a little more.

TIGHT CALVES

Tight calves are common because they're doing so much work. They're involved in the landing phase but also the propulsion phase.

The question is, why are they tight? Tightness is the result of something else going on; it might be a positional thing, however, more often with runners it's a weakness. The calf simply doesn't have the strength needed to do what you're asking of it.

The test for this is normal calf raises. The general population should be able to do 21 calf raises on a single leg (guys can do slightly more at 24), so that's the starting point to aim for. Do this off a step a couple of times a week and progressively add some weight. During running the calf has to deal with nearly five times your bodyweight of pressure. Working up towards that number is the simplest way to safeguard against pain long-term.

THE FIXES

There are more general ways to prevent injury, one of the most popular being sports massages. Are they a luxury or necessity? Well, it depends on the runner. There was an excellent research paper that came out last year[26] that compared a lot of recovery techniques and massage came out on top. It won for reducing delayed onset muscle soreness (DOMS) and lowering perceived fatigue. And so, if you find it helps, then it's a necessity. If you find you don't need it and that you can bounce back to do your next run without it, then don't worry – save your money!

Performance to my mind is fitness minus fatigue, so if you want to perform – especially injury-free – then you need to recover, and it's down to the runner to find out what works for them. But for me, the most important thing that I've learned about avoiding injury is to take sleep more seriously. It's the single greatest tool in your arsenal when protecting your muscles and joints from the rigours of a new passion for running.

And lastly, don't panic if you miss a run. You'll only end up squeezing it in and probably overwork yourself, which can cause an injury. Running should be fun and if you're doing it as part of a new, healthy habit, build up to it slowly. For success over the years to come, not just resolutions, less is often more.

On The Run With . . . Esmée Gummer

When Esmée went in for routine surgery she didn't expect to leave the hospital paralysed from the waist down. Over the past decade she has learned to walk again, rebuild her physical and mental strength, and today she has marathon and ultra-marathon medals in her collection. That, ladies and gentlemen, is what you call a comeback. This is her story.

AL: For anyone who was to meet you for the first time today, you'd be a picture of health and, in many ways I suppose, you absolutely are. You're at the forefront of the London fitness scene, helping other people to reach their own goals. Life, it seems, has worked out great. But that was in no way guaranteed – in fact, not so long ago you couldn't even walk. People talk about having a fitness journey, but yours has been exactly that!

EG: Yes, you're so right. I grew up dancing and had planned to go to dance college when I suffered from a hernia. I needed to have it repaired so went in for a routine operation to fix it. But during the procedure I had a reaction to either the anaesthetic or the anti-sickness drugs and I seizured for 8 hours – it left me paralysed from the waist down.

It was strange really. The first three days I was completely out of it, my speech wasn't there, neither was my short-term memory. So it was a strange way to come to terms with it because I didn't just wake up suddenly and say, 'Oh my god, I'm paralysed.' The only way to describe it is like when you're drunk and you can feel yourself sobering up slowly – there was no shock moment.

I was in the hospital for three weeks doing rehab. Mentally I was totally with it but I couldn't walk. When they let me leave the hospital I could put one leg in front of the other – just – but I still needed a wheelchair most of the time. My rehab process was nowhere near finished.

AL: What was the message from the doctors when you were wheeled out of the hospital?

EG: There was a crucial moment when the doctor did say that I wasn't going to walk again, and I understand why he said it. It's because my speech came back, and my short-term memory returned, but then from the waist down my recovery stalled. Normally, your body heals in a progressive way, but after day six it just stopped healing at my waist. That was the moment where he said, 'This is it.'

AL: But you strike me as the type of person who wasn't just going to accept this fate. Was there a moment where you decided that the doctor was wrong?

EG: Do you know what? Yes. And it might sound cheesy but I just knew that I was going to be able to walk again. I just knew that it wasn't the final word for me and I was going to make certain of it.

AL: Did the recovery process take a long time?

EG: Yes, but it was the mental side that took longer. It completely knocked my confidence. That took years to recover. I was so insecure, and I didn't believe in myself. And I started having to deal with an emotion that I hadn't experienced before, and that was resentment and jealousy against people. Especially against those doing what I wanted to do, especially dancers.

I had a group of friends at dance school and we'd trained together there specifically to go away to college. That was the goal. And at 18 they all left without me. I couldn't even look at them or like their pictures on Facebook despite the fact I should have been supporting them as my friends. And I hate that. My mum always raised me to use jealousy and competition in a healthy way.

AL: It's understandable, the frustration must have been unreal. But you soon turned your attention to supporting others in a different way – when was it you decided you wanted to become a PT? A brave move for someone with such a bad injury, I've got to say!

EG: I was actually eligible for a disability allowance that meant I wouldn't have to work while I was recovering. However, my brother is disabled because he has learning difficulties and he *can't* work, but he would do anything to be able to. I thought, I can't take the allowance, because my brain is all there I can do everything, I just can't walk.

I took an office job so that I could sit down all day. But while I was sat there I decided that I wanted to get into fitness because fitness had not only helped me to recover physically but I'd also learned so much about training the mind and how a strong mind can benefit your life outside of the gym. So I took the qualification online and waited until I was able to do the physical part of the testing. Then I went straight to a gym to get a job and do the level 3 PT qualification. The thought process was pretty simple: if I can motivate myself to recover from paralysis, then I can motivate someone to do a push-up.

AL: And you can definitely motivate people to do a push-up, I've seen you in action! Since then your career has gone from strength to strength and you now train a number of celebrity clients, but you reached a milestone in your own personal fitness journey when you toed the line of the London marathon. I remember seeing you in the start pen and you saying that you couldn't believe you were there because at one point you were never going to be able to walk again. But there you were about to tackle 26.2 . . .

EG: Ah, you're giving me goosebumps just thinking about it! That experience was obviously incredibly personal for me after being told I'd never run again. I actually managed my first run a year after I got paralysed. I used to run all the time, I did 5k before school as a kid, I loved it – but then out on my first run, my right leg went dead. I remember thinking, I can't believe this is happening. I'd made it a kilometre. And so, I just said to myself, I've not come this far to deal with another problem and I can do everything else, if I can't run then I just won't do it ever again. So, I just gave up running. I was defeated.

A few years passed and then a year before the 2018 marathon – I didn't have a spot then – I just started running. My mum said to me, if you can teach yourself to walk again, then you can teach yourself to run. I just got out there and started moving. I made a mental note that if my leg went dead then that was no longer enough to make me quit and I was going to keep going. Then, out of the blue, I was offered a spot on a marathon team. I'd only been running for about six months, and I sat there looking at my phone contemplating it, and then just went: 'Well, I guess this is happening!'

AL: So you really were a beginner all over again when it came to training for the marathon start line?

EG: Absolutely! I hadn't run properly for seven years! But then I began training the January before the race. I was determined. I had it in my head that if I could complete a marathon then I was no longer paralysed. It was going to be a character change for me.

It wasn't easy. There were runs that I'd get part of the way through and have to get a taxi home. I remember one where I was doing 18 miles and my leg went dead – it was about two weeks before the marathon and I was out with a friend who had to piggyback me to the taxi.

By going dead I mean that I couldn't drive it at all. I couldn't lift the knee. Once I sat down afterwards, it was worse. That was devastating. And it stayed dead for three days after. I remember that even when getting into the car I had to physically lift in in with me. I admit, my confidence was absolutely shot. But I couldn't give up. Movement returned and I just thought: 'Well, I'm going to get round no matter what – if I walk the marathon, then I walk it.'

And you'll know this, Amy, there are always people who ask, 'Oh, what time did you get?' But I never wanted it to be like that. There's part of you that wants to say, I got this time, but I also have all these excuses as to why that's the case. But no, I wanted to cross the line with my head held high. And that's what people should do – they shouldn't worry about what other people think of their time because nobody knows what they've gone through to get there. And, more importantly, they don't need to. It's your story.

AL: You've gone on to run more marathons and even an ultra . . .

EG: I can't even believe that I am able to say I ran 250k across the Wadi Rum desert in Jordan. But life is amazing, you've just got to be prepared to be uncomfortable sometimes in return for the wonder of the world. And, I'm totally hooked [on running] now. I've learned to love that feeling of being in pain – suffering through it but coming out the other end. That sense of accomplishment is so amazing. That's why exercise is so incredible; you can willingly put yourself into a vulnerable position, try something that's uncomfortable and see how far you can go and what you can learn about yourself. People shouldn't exercise to get six-packs, they should exercise to learn about themselves, because the more you know about yourself the more you can use that in day-to-day life.

Your Chapter 7 Action Plan

- Listen to pain and don't grit your teeth through it. It'll only leave you with wine coolers wrapped around your shins

- Track your weekly mileage and be careful how quickly you add distance. Remember the 10 per cent rule!

- Don't let injuries leave you sofa-bound. If there's stuff you can do pain-free, do that, and use it as the starting point of your rehab

- Test your calf strength. Aim for 20 reps as a baseline for single-leg calf raises and then start adding weight

- Book yourself in for a sports massage and see if it powers up your next run. Go on, treat yourself . . .

CHAPTER 8

Girl Bossing It

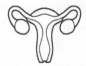

My Journey

For years my period was a problem, and one I chose to deal with in private. But as more and more women progress to the top of their sports, periods and their impact on performance are finally becoming part of the conversation. In fact, the bleeding edge of science thinks your period could help you to go even faster.

There's a quote that regularly pops up on my Instagram feed. It reads: 'When women support each other incredible things happen.' And though it's one thing to post it and quite another to actually live by it, I truly feel like a seachange towards female success and empowerment is in full flow.

In Iceland, women ensured they had the final say on the gender pay gap with a law that fines companies who pay men and women in the same job differently; in Saudia Arabia a ban on women driving has finally been reversed (although there's still plenty of work to do in that country, obviously); and in

Lebanon female activists forced parliament to repeal an ancient law that *still* allowed male rapists to be exonerated if they married their victims. What progress looks like differs around the world, and while some glass ceilings have been shattered, others remain intact. But progress marches on. Importantly, in Britain today women can have multi-hyphen titles with wife and mother now just two options, not obligations.

One shining light for women has been their progress in professional sport. Across a myriad of disciplines, women haven't just raised the game but are blazing trails that leave their male counterparts eating dust. The sport of ultra-running is one where women are excelling beyond expectations. Not only are female runners clocking times faster than their male competition, they're exhibiting an inner strength that men might never be able to achieve.

At 2019's Spine Race – arguably one of the UK's (if not the world's) toughest runs – there were two front runners, Jasmin Paris and Eugeni Roselló Solé. The course covers a distance of more than 10 marathons and ascends a total elevation equivalent to one and a half Everests. Three-quarters of the way through the race, things changed. Roselló Solé, a former champion, was forced to seek medical advice and chose to use the time to catch some much-needed rest. Paris saw an opportunity. She made the decision to forgo a proper rest stop and only paused to eat and express breast milk for her daughter before carrying on. She stormed to victory. Roselló Solé eventually crashed out 4 miles before the finish through injury, and the next runner wouldn't cross the finish line for another 15 hours. Paris' performance has been hailed as 'extraordinary' and 'a run of a lifetime', but in the ultra-endurance world this calibre of female excellence is no anomaly. In 2019, ultra-cyclist Fiona Kolbinger became the first woman to win the Transcontinental

Race. Her victory over 4,200k was made all the more remarkable by the fact that it was her first race and her next closest opponent was 10 hours behind her.

The supporting science behind a theory that women having a genetic advantage in endurance races is still in its infancy, but the rationale is there. Women have a greater distribution of slow-twitch muscle fibres and superior emotional coping strategies. It's only with the advent of these new, extreme endurance events that women's innate grit has been thrown into the spotlight. Over shorter distances like the marathon, the difference between the world record times for men and women is big, at over 12 minutes. For women to catch up it would require running at a mile pace that's around half a minute faster. When you're already running nearly a 5-minute mile, that's not easy. In fact, some believe it's near impossible because women don't possess the strength, lung size and aerobic power that men do. However, when you extend the competition to runs from anything between 5 and 100 hours, the benefits of bigger lungs and legs peter out. It's then that a woman's mental mettle comes to the fore.

And not even women's other superpower, giving birth, can slow us down. Ultra-marathon runner Sophie Power is an example of this. While running the infamously tough 105-mile Ultra-Trail du Mont Blanc (UTMB), Power stopped to breastfeed her then three-month-old son, Cormac. The moment was caught on camera and before Power knew it, her breasts had started a global debate: what are women capable of postpartum? And is it selfish to prioritise the miles of racing over motherhood?

Power isn't the only runner juggling the marathon of motherhood with marathons of miles while either pregnant or postpartum. On social media #pregnantrunners are not only expanding in body but in numbers too. There are mums running half marathons mid-term and achieving times not far off their pre-pregnancy pace, and women traversing mountains between breastfeeds.

Outside of endurance sports there are more awe-inspiring stories. Perhaps the most famous is Dame Jessica Ennis-Hill winning gold in the heptathlon in Beijing only nine months after having her son Reggie. Even Ennis-Hill was surprised by her success: 'I'm still shocked to this day that I was able to come back from having my son, go back into training and then win the world championships,' she told me.

The belief that a post-baby body will no longer perform how it used to is outdated. In fact, Power states that part of her success in endurance sports is linked to the fact that as a mum she is permanently sleep-deprived. Unlike other athletes who are used to their comfy eight hours, Power has learned to function on a lot less, so a night of UTMB is little different to the broken sleep of nighttime feeds and nappy changes. She just runs with it.

And so the picture of women crossing the finish line to collect their medal with one hand and carrying their baby with the other proves that women are just as strong as men. In many ways they are stronger. But that doesn't mean we're equal. Women are different, and ignoring that fact of biology can cause problems, especially when you're active.

What I'm referring to, of course, is that time of the month. That time when a woman can be doubled over with period pain, cuddling a hot-water bottle like the Care Bear from their youth. There are numerous names and euphemisms for female menstruation: Aunt Flow, on the rag, lady business, crimson tide – but just because we have so many ways to describe it doesn't mean we're OK talking about it. Recent research[27] hinted that as many as 82 per cent of female athletes are not discussing their monthly cycles with their coach. And it's this period taboo that is causing some sportswomen to suffer.

A few years ago British tennis player Heather Watson attributed her loss in the Australian Open to her monthly cycle. Her 'girls' problems' did not serve her well that day and she went out on the court with nausea and low energy, set up to fail. And she's not the only one. British runner Jess Judd has previously admitted that her menstrual cycle can be the difference between her placing first and last. But why?

Each month the female body goes through a number of changes as it prepares to play host to your potential offspring. If your female parts were a holiday it would look a little like this. Imagine your ovaries are the destination airport. When you (the egg) land, they call you an Uber (your fallopian tubes). Your Uber arrives at the airport, you happily jump in and head to your hotel (your womb). Sometimes, while en route you might bump into another holidaymaker (the sperm) and if you guys hit it off, then you're in for a totally different ride. When you reach your hotel in the womb you'll bed down and stay on your extended holiday, only leaving when you've outgrown your surroundings (a bit like when you've eaten every item on the all-inclusive menu). If your Uber didn't bump into pals en route then your break will be cut short. No womb hotel for you, missy. You're leaving along with all the shower gel and slipper freebies you can take (womb lining) to head out through the front door. And that's that. Period.

This monthly cycle is powered by hormones, which increase and decrease depending on what physiological changes need to happen. That means, unlike a man's body that is pretty stable from day-to-day, yours isn't. Your internal environment is in flux and this causes more side effects than just periods. But we learn incredibly little about this complex biology. In school, we're too busy tittering at rolling a condom on to a cucumber to take notice of the ins and outs of our reproductive cycle. And though I'm no scientist, I've made it my mission to educate myself, especially when it comes to running.

Periods and performance

The obvious effect of having to deal with a period while exercising is the annoyance of, well, having to deal with it. It's a fact highlighted by Kiran Gandhi, who in 2015 decided to bleed freely while running the London Marathon. Her rationale? A sanitary towel might chafe and wearing a tampon could require a portaloo pitstop to change it. Neither were favourable options for Gandhi, so she ran *sans* sanitary products. Aside from getting people talking, this radical move opened up the conversation: how should women deal with the realities of menstruation while exercising?

Menstrual symptoms that can affect training:

- Feeling bloated

- Breast tenderness

- Mood swings

- Feeling irritable

- Period pain

- Low energy

- Broken sleep

- Food cravings

In a large study led by a team of researchers from St Mary's University[28] for FitrWoman, over 70 per cent of women surveyed reported receiving no education about the relationship between their period and exercise. Which is a problem. Separate research suggests that there is a link between female hormones and knee injuries. In fact, women are four to six times more likely to tear their ACL than men. This is because the menstrual cycle can make joints and ligaments loosen. Being on the pill can help to prevent this, but it's by no means a cure-all. Athletes such as Paula Radcliffe have been quick to argue that playing God with Mother Nature might not be so much of a good thing. Over the years she has been vocal about her negative experience with norethisterone; a drug used to delay menstruation. While it stopped her bleeding it didn't relieve the other issues associated with menstruation.

In my own case it's hard to know which came first in my life: PCOS or bulimia – science says there's a two-way relationship between them. Maybe one of them is to blame for my experience of amenorrhea (no periods) or maybe both played a part, but unlike Radcliffe, I didn't ask for my body to put menstruation on hold. It just did it. My uterus decided that due to overexercising and underfuelling, it was not in a fit state to care for a baby. At the time, 20-something me only saw the wins of this situation: no need to buy sanitary products or spray white sheets with Vanish to remove smears of period blood. But my body was rebelling.

Along with no periods I suffered from excess body hair, random pelvic pain and hormonal acne. I still have scars from the latter today. But the big kicker came when the doctor informed me that I was at risk of osteoporosis. My oestrogen had dropped to the same level as women going through menopause and I was now at risk of weak bones. I was sent for bone-density scans and put on calcium tablets that looked more like horse supplements they were so big. The fact that this happened and I didn't tell anyone about it is telling of the times I grew up in. Thankfully my body and the conversation surrounding menstruation have moved on. Thirty-something me is an open book on my body, because talking about periods should be as normal as having them. Globally, 300 million women are on their period at any one time. That's 300 million women who could be using their cycle for success. Yes, with some smart scheduling you can actually turn your period into a performance-enhancer. You just need a little help from this chapter's expert . . .

'I'm working on
myself,
for myself,
by myself'

Follow The Leader

Georgie Bruvinels is a research scientist and driving force of the @fitrwoman project – an app that helps you track your menstrual cycle and provides personalised training and nutritional sugges-tions tailored to the changing hormone levels throughout your life. She's a pioneer of ensuring women can train in a way that really benefits them, and it's working. She worked closely with the US women's football team on their way to World Cup glory and has recently been signed by Chelsea to share her expertise. And now she wants to help you, too.

INTO THE UNKNOWN

It's incredible how much we truly don't know about the female body. We know even less than you might imagine, and the reason is fascinating – if also frustrating. If you go back into the history books, around the time of the First and Second World Wars, it was decided that scientific and medical research shouldn't be conducted in women at all. There were concerns about doing tests on women who may be carrying unborn children – testing and scanning for pregnancy was obviously far harder back then. Incredibly, this was followed blindly until the 70s.

In the US, the Office of National Research on Women's Health finally announced this was crazy and something needed to be done. Eventually in the 90s there was a law passed that said researchers actually *had* to do research in women. You could no longer put a drug on the market, for example, without having first done research in women. Even now, 80 per cent of drugs are withdrawn from the market because of side effects on women, because they simply weren't checked initially.

The problem comes because, as a researcher, you want to find the next big thing and want to understand the cutting edge of research. You want to be at the forefront and you do that by working with men, because the background research has already been done. As a result, a lot of female physiology remains relatively unknown.

Closing that gender research gap is one of my missions. But that's easier said than done. People don't want to talk about their menstrual cycles, for one. The taboo still exists. We're trying to change that but it won't happen overnight. There are also other considerations like the impact of hormonal contraception, for example. Or testing on people with irregular cycles or dysfunction. There is research going on but so much more is needed.

THE IMPORTANCE OF TRACKING

A large part of my agenda is inspiring women to look after themselves and understand themselves. You should not be in a position where you just have to accept, 'Oh well, I'm just not happy today.' There's always a cause, and getting to know yourself through tracking, in particular your cycle, which plays such a large part in the release of hormones, can arm you with the knowledge to both understand and take action.

Understanding your body builds confidence and it also makes getting help far easier. If you're suddenly spotting loads, or if you've skipped a cycle or you're experiencing new symptoms and they don't feel quite right, then you are able to walk into your GP surgery and say: 'Actually, I've been tracking my cycle and this is what I found,' – that's a game changer because they can start helping you right away.

THE CASE FOR KNOWING YOUR CYCLE

Firstly, it's really important that women are menstruating for optimum health. And so that is the first, most obvious thing to check. Secondly, we have done some research now; we surveyed 14,000 women,[29] and found that more than 80 per cent experience symptoms (e.g. menstrual cramps) every single cycle. If that many are experiencing symptoms every cycle, added to the fact that 93 per cent of them say that those symptoms hold them back and prevent them from performing optimally, then it's obvious that a plan needs to be put in place to help people manage it.

A plan allows you to take the initiative and attempt to reduce symptoms at the right time, but also it's worth considering whether a plan could be used to turn your menstrual cycle into a training aid. Do you perform better, recover faster, eat better during certain phases of the cycle? Fascinatingly, the answer to most of those is, yes. We know in the first couple of phases you adapt and respond to the separate points of strength training better. The implications there being that if you focus on doing your heavy weight work in the first two weeks of the cycle then you can train more effectively and improve more quickly.

Equally, it's really important to work with your menstrual cycle to help you manage your own expectations. As women we can be really hard on ourselves, but if we work with our cycle we may understand the comedowns better and be easier on ourselves. You may be running but find it impossible to get in a rhythm and struggle all the way around. You may spend a week struggling for the motivation to get up early for that workout class. You may suddenly be really, really hungry and dying for a sugar binge. All of these have internal factors at play.

There are other, more serious considerations, too. From an injury-risk perspective we know that in the first half of the cycle, up to the ovulation point, women are more prone to certain injury types because their biomechanics change, and their ligaments become more susceptible to injury. Inflammation rises, or if you have a history of a lax ankle then that comes into play. I, for example, am really good at rolling my ankles! And I'm more susceptible to that at certain points in my cycle. There are so many considerations, that when armed with the knowledge you can both prime and protect yourself during different phases.

HOW TO MATCH YOUR TRAINING TO YOUR CYCLE

Each phase vaguely corresponds to a week of your cycle. No two women are the same, so remember to listen to your body, but the guidelines below should help you to adapt your sessions as your cycle progresses.

Phase 1
This begins with the start of menstruation. At this time your body is primed for you to hit the gym and to shift the emphasis of your training to muscle and strength – your ability to adapt is at its peak. Though don't get ahead of yourself; increase loads gradually to avoid injury. There is increasing evidence to suggest that neuromuscular control is lower, making you more susceptible to painful tweaks, so focus on activations now, too (refresh your memory of these by revisiting Chapter 5). Exercise during this time will also release feel-good endorphins to help with potential cramps.

Phase 2

Intense sessions and strength training can still form a major part of your training during this phase, too. In fact, you may want to go all-in as your energy levels will also spike, meaning you'll struggle less with the motivation to get to the gym and train. You can up the intensity of your recovery, too. Your pain threshold is higher now and that means an intense date with a foam roller or massage therapist will be made more manageable. Just remember: this extra training load requires lots of sleep to maximise the benefits.

Phase 3

This phase begins with ovulation (around day 14 for most women). Slow down on the free weights and switch the emphasis to your long runs. Research suggests that your endurance will peak this week, so make the most of it and up the distance because you'll find it easier. That said, overall energy may start to wane – in which case, lower the intensity (e.g. pace) while maintaining the overall distance or time. As energy begins to drop so does power, so take that as a signal to take your foot off the gas in the gym too, either by reducing the sets or reps. Use that extra time for another few minutes of mobility work. Again, Chapter 5 can help you here.

Phase 4

In the final week of your cycle, as you head towards menstruation, symptoms of pre-menstrual stress may well be in full swing. Though you may not be in the mood, maintaining your training schedule will help with symptoms. HIIT will help in the short term by producing mood-elevating endorphins, but I would prefer to recommend adding in yoga and Pilates as a more sustainable fix. These low-intensity pursuits have been linked to successfully easing stress levels.

HOW TO MATCH YOUR NUTRITION PLAN TO YOUR CYCLE, TOO

Phase 1

During menstruation, inflammation levels are at their highest while our hormone levels are at an all-time low. White blood cells and your immune system are down too – so you need to be mindful of illness. Boosting your iron levels with extra portions of leafy green veg, beef and beans will help there. Anti-inflammatory foods are a smart and simple addition to your shopping list, too. Foods rich in omega-3s like flaxseeds and chia seeds, berries, oily fish and walnuts can alleviate symptoms. As a positive, your body's ability to metabolise carbs for fuel is running high, so tuck in before your most difficult sessions.

Phase 2

Your energy levels will gradually begin to increase when menstruation ends, as your oestrogen levels rise but your proges-terone level stays very low. As you now know, this means you can train harder, but it'll only work if you adapt your diet to support these endeavours. Extra collagen from berries, almonds and avocados will aid soft-tissue recovery, plus the extra vitamin C in the berries will also help with muscle, tendon and ligament recovery. This one is more obvious, but ensuring you top up your protein levels with eggs, cottage cheese, peanut butter or chicken is also a smart idea.

Phase 3

This one can get a little tricky as you may end up feeling less strong and therefore train less hard, but then also feel more hungry. You'll therefore need to be mindful of overeating. Eating more fibre at mealtimes to keep blood-sugar levels stable will help. Right now your body is using fats as its main energy source, so keep oily fish, seeds and avocados at the top of your shopping list. However, that doesn't mean you should neglect the mid-run carbs on runs over an hour. Muscle breakdown may also increase, but a protein-rich snack within 30-minutes of your run will stop this developing into extra soreness.

Phase 4
The effects of PMS (pre-menstrual syndrome) begin to kick in as hormones decline sharply and the inflammatory response goes into overdrive, causing PMS symptoms. The fruit, eggs, nuts and other foods high in anti-inflammatories mentioned before will continue to help reduce symptoms. Those high in saturated fats, however, may worsen symptoms. If you feel yourself getting hungry between meals, counter cravings with slow-release carbs that are higher in fibre, such as sweet potato, and if you're not sleeping, then try foods rich in melatonin, like bananas and oats.

IT'S ALL IN YOUR HEAD

Getting your mind on side can also help to minimise the negative symptoms of your cycle. I work with the US women's soccer team who recently partnered with the meditation app Headspace. Some of the players found it game-changing. One team member was regularly missing two days a month of training due to menstrual cycle symptoms, then a new meditation and mindfulness habit suddenly made the whole experience a lot more manageable.

We know that psychological elements can exacerbate symptoms. If you're psychologically stressed, if you're going through a difficult time at work or at home, exam stresses, anything – we know that it can affect your cycle to either elongate it or make symptoms worse, so any way of mitigating that is really powerful. And 15 minutes of meditation on your commute may be your solution.

IMPERFECT TIMING

And finally, we know that it's coming every month, but that timing doesn't always play ball when it concerns the events and competitions you're training for. But if you've been tracking and you know that your next 10k falls on the date when your symptoms are at their worst, that doesn't mean you need to throw in the towel.

My approach would be to try and understand your cycle, and put in a strategy to offset the negative effects. If you experience really bad premenstrual symptoms, what are they? If you experience really bad nausea, or you get migraines, then they're probably inflammation-driven. And that means having a few days of taking an anti-inflammatory like ibuprofen or simply increasing your fish intake. The fatty acids in a portion of salmon can help to curb inflammation that's driving symptoms. We know that psychological stress can bring up those symptoms too, so work out what you can do to moderate that. It may mean delegating more jobs at work or reducing your training load. If you're craving food constantly at a certain time, split your day up so that you're having five meals a day, not three, and keeping energy levels stable in the run-up to an event. As I've mentioned, it's individual to you but there are usually solutions to whatever your cycle throws at you.

On The Run With . . . Tina Muir

For most, being able to make your running habit stick is the primary concern. Not so Tina Muir. A professional runner who has dedicated herself to the sport since the age of 14, Muir's PBs speak for themselves: from a 16:08 5k through to a 2:36 marathon. But that dedication takes a toll, and now Muir is leading the pack in raising awareness of amenorrhea (no periods). She's released a book, Overcoming Amenorrhea, *and is a leading light, championing the importance of understanding the relationship between exercise and your menstrual cycle, especially if you have hopes of starting a family. I caught up with Muir to hear her story.*

AL: A lot of people might not know that, despite being a GB athlete, you're based in the US. How long have you been over there now?

TM: About 14 years. It's weird to think that I've now been in America for longer than I was in England.

AL: And was it your running that took you to the US?

TM: Yes, for university. But I started running back in the UK. I always tell the story that at school I would hide from cross-country trials in the toilets because I had no interest. And then at the age of 14, I have no idea what caused the turnaround, it almost feels like I blacked out, but I essentially woke up from that blackout and was on the cross-country team. One of the teachers said to my parents that I had a talent for it and that they should take me to a running club, and so that's what we did. I went to a club in the next town along, met my coach and went from there.

AL: Did you stay with your first coach?

TM: Yes, and I credit my success to him. As a kid I wanted to push myself harder and do more. I wanted to win races and to compete with the best, but he kept saying that he wanted me to have a life-long career and, crucially, that he didn't want to push me too hard when I was still growing up. He kept saying the best is yet to come. And by doing that he managed to still keep me upbeat and excited and wanting to do well in races, but also held me back enough so that I could be my best in my early 20s. There are so many who start getting serious at 14 and are then already burned out by 16 or 18. I've passed that lesson on to as many people as possible to make sure that people know that the most important thing is to have fun with running, especially when you are a teenager.

AL: And did you manage to follow those rules and not sneak off to do extra?

TM: I didn't sneak off, no. But it meant that I really pushed myself. I always had an ability to take things to a new level, and when he gave me something to do I would always max out. Plus, I make a point of always listening to my coaches when they tell me a hard No. I remember when I was training with my husband as my coach and the most mileage I ever did was 99.7 miles in a week. And I asked him if I could go out and do that last 0.3 to hit 100, just that once. His answer was a flat no and so I didn't. I'm good at sticking to it.

AL: That capacity for hard work is amazing. But it comes with risks. How long was it until you realised that that running was taking a toll on your body and playing with your cycle?

TM: I lost my period when I was still in England and about 18 years old – I lost it for a few months. I remember I was trying to find more people who were running my distance to train with, and so I went to go and run with Paula Radcliffe's coach. It was really intense. That's when I lost my period. It put me into the oversimplified mindset that it was just down to hard training. Rather than it being about nutrition or fuelling myself properly. And so I just assumed that every time I trained really hard that I was going to lose my period.

After university I went for a gap year, took time off from training and my period came back and was really regular. But then when I started training again it started to really mess around. Unfortunately, and extremely unhelpfully, I was told by someone that I should lose weight to help with my performance. I believed them and then after that my period completely stopped. I went to see a specialist about it and basically all their advice boiled down to was that you need to stop running and it'll come back.

AL: And at the time that was a no-go?

TM: I remember going back to England and going to the doctor and she asked when my last period was. I told her it was years ago and she again said it'll come back when I stopped running. I then told her, well, I can't stop running for at least another five years, and she just couldn't understand why that was. But to me running was my job. Running was paying for my housing. It was paying for my degree. It paid for everything. And so I couldn't give it up, even if it meant messing my body up for a few years. At that point I was willing to take the risk.

AL: Was it something that played on your mind day-to-day?

TM: No, and I think that was simply because I was in my mid-20s, and falling pregnant was the last thing that I wanted. And so it was easy to push it out of my mind because I reasoned that the only time to really care was when I was ready to have a child. Now I know that's not right and not good, but at the time that's how I rationalised it. However, when I was around women and they were talking about running with cramps or general chat around periods I would feel ashamed and slink out of the room because I didn't want people to ask me.

Doctors would always ask me when my last period was and I couldn't give them the answer. That was embarrassing. But it was also so easy for me to say, 'Oh I'll deal with that next month, I'm really busy this month so I'll sort that out next month.' Having had all the medical checks, and them telling me that there was nothing wrong with me internally, then it became easy for me to simply start brushing it under the carpet.

AL: Did they check you for PCOS?

TM: Yes, so I had all kinds of tests like ultrasounds. They put me on a really strong hormone that did get me to have a period, and it was one of the most painful experiences of my life. And that kind of proved the point that I can have a period but I'm just not because of the running. And so that was just more reason to let it go.

But then as I came to the end of my professional running career in my late 20s, I started to think about other things. Firstly, becoming a mother and that being the kickstart, but also the more basic fact that living like that wasn't right. I felt I was hiding this big lie. It's OK to say that something isn't working for a couple of years (although it's not really) but when you then start getting up to 5, 6, 7, 8 years with a crucial part of you not working, then I started to realise it was a problem.

From then on I was constantly trying to change things to help. I tried adding more fats to my diet. I tried eating more 'clean' ingredients. Eating more protein. I tried getting acupuncture. I got a urine test. I tried everything but it all just kept coming back saying that I was good and healthy.

AL: And at the time were you still running crazy high mileage?

TM: Interestingly, at the time I lost my period initially I was probably running the same mileage as I'm running right now. And now I have my period regularly. Back then, however, I had that one coach telling me that I should lose weight, and so began a time of restriction. Essentially I got into a negative mindset of having to earn my food. I wasn't starving myself by any means, but the dangerous thing that a lot of women fall into is this kind of grey zone that I was in. You're not starving yourself but you're not eating enough, you're eating just the amount that you need to function.

The crazy thing is that you can then start to see the side effects as an advantage. For example, my eyes would ping open at 4am at this time. And I thought that was great. I could get more done in a day. But now, rightly, I see that as my body being on edge. And that was down to restriction. If I did a long run I felt that I had earned a massive meal. And I would go out and eat a lot and people would say, 'Wow you're eating so much.' But on the other days where I was only running for an hour I would eat much healthier and closer to the line.

AL: What did you change in your diet that made the change in your body for your periods to return?

TM: No one thing helped, it was just a case of eating more. And the easiest way to do that was simply to eat the things that I enjoyed most. That's cakes and pancakes. That was the quickest way for me to do it. Obviously in terms of long-term health it's better to do it through healthy ingredients, but when you've lost your period for years and you want it back ASAP, and it's a case of not eating enough calories or getting enough calories through eating traditionally unhealthy foods, then it became a case of getting those calories, no matter how. Yes, the type of calories matter – if you don't eat enough healthy fats then you're going to have trouble, for example – but really it's about consuming more energy for your body.

AL: And obviously it worked!

TM: Yes, but I'm the quickest to say that I do not have a blueprint for how to go from not having a period to getting pregnant. I was incredibly lucky that it happened so quickly for me, but I don't want that to provide some form of false hope for people out there that it's going to be simple.

AL: Were you surprised yourself?

TM: Yes and no. I went all in. I ate all the food I needed to eat and I truly rested, which I'd never really done before. I put my feet up on the couch. I got massages and acupuncture. I did everything I could to get into the right place and get my period back.

AL: Did you feel different mentally as well as physically? When I've taken time off from the stress of training a weight is lifted from my mind, too. Or as an athlete did you struggle to adjust to not doing what you'd done for so long?

TM: I think I found it easier than I expected. I thought that I was going to struggle to be around the sport and do anything in the sport without competing. But I was starting a business to help people in the sport and so that allowed me to be supportive and happy for other people doing well, not just myself.

I realise a lot of that contentment came down to it being my choice. When you have an injury and the sport is taken from you, that can be hard. But this was my choice. I made the decision to stop. I made the decision to get my period back. I chose to have a family. And I think the clarity I got from making that decision helped in so many other ways mentally, too.

Before then I had insomnia and I would be up at 4am, but now I sleep well and I enjoy sleep. I can fall asleep quickly and I don't feel that constant low level of anxiety in the background that I did before. Stepping back gave me that space I needed to realise that I am not my accomplishments.

AL: You made the difficult decision to leave running for the sake of yourself and starting a family, and now you're back running again about a year after having a kid. What are you doing differently?

TM: I've run a half marathon but I'm not training anywhere near the level I was before, and I don't have the desire to, either. And I don't know if I ever will. I like to think that there will come a time where I can run again for another GB vest, but that's not what I'm interested in right now. Right now it's about running for joy. If I wake up and I don't feel good, I don't run. And if I miss a couple of runs in a row because I'm too busy then so be it. I remember that running doesn't have to be about committing to these massive goals, you can come at it at all levels. You can go through periods of being totally committed but you can also go through other stages where you're just out to enjoy it, to explore scenery and to make friends.

AL: And are you tracking your cycle?

TM: Yes! It's funny but I do still get excited when I get my period simply because I went all those years without getting it. Also because I've breastfed for over a year, it took a while for it to come back after giving birth, too. Really I'm still only on period 6, 7, 8, so it still feels kind of new to me. It's like being 14 all over again.

> **Your Chapter 8 Action Plan**
>
> - Break the taboo. Periods are a fact of women's lives, so get comfortable talking about them
>
> - Start tracking your cycle and arm yourself with all the knowledge you need, plus a headstart if you ever need to go to the GP with a problem
>
> - Focus your strength training on the first half of your cycle
>
> - Be extra careful to protect against injury at the end of your cycle by being diligent with your warm-up protocols
>
> - Look at your symptoms and deal with them individually; for nausea eat anti-inflammatory foods, for cravings eat more, smaller meals

CHAPTER 9

Thinking On Your Feet

My Journey

The mind can be a hindrance or a help on your running journey. Equally, running can be the help you need to feel mentally stronger and more resilient than ever before. Life is full of ups and downs but I've found that mastering the correct mindset can help to keep me moving forward.

When I was a child I never felt like an outsider. It didn't matter that in the space of 10 years I moved house nearly every year, racking up more 'previous addresses' than a fraudster on the run. I was confident and outgoing and never failed to make friends. Even during secondary school when I fell out with, or outgrew friendships, I was never alone. Not really. Within a week or two I'd found common ground with another person or two, and embraced opening my world to new voices, thoughts and lifestyles. At university, the need to forge new friendships once again presented itself and I reignited a youthful interest in netball. Doing so helped me befriend the president of the netball team and her squad of pals. At the time, Facebook hadn't long launched and to do this day, I remember when my 'Friends' count topped 500. According to the internet, I had *a lot* of friends.

Around this time, however, I was also caught up in a toxic on-off relationship. We'd met in this first year of university and I dove headfirst into coupledom, choosing to spend time with him and his friends at the expense of nights out with mine (either new or pals back home). For a couple of years I would head to Croydon to hang out with him and his social circle, and although I was committed to this situation, according to the folder of screenshots of other women on his computer, he wasn't. We would regularly fight and I'd be left emotional and empty with few people I felt I could actually lean on. Understandably, you forgo the privilege of snotty, blubbery telephone conversations with friends when you've failed to check in with how they are in a long time. I accept that to only phone when in need is not true friendship. And so, after years of feeling secure in my social circles, I was left with plenty of friends on social media, but feeling like an outsider in many of those relationships.

According to the BBC's Loneliness Experiment,[30] I wasn't the only one. Of the group that they surveyed for this project 40 per cent of 16–24-year-olds reported feeling lonely often or very often. Plus, those who felt lonely had more 'online only' Facebook friends. So, as much as the internet has opened doors, it has also closed them. But it's not just younger men and women who report this. Research by the Co-op and British Red Cross[31] reported that 9 million people identify with feeling 'lonely', prompting the government to confront this epidemic by appointing Tracey Crouch as the UK's first loneliness minister. But, how do you deal with something that is so difficult to define? Loneliness, unlike tendonitis or a sprained ankle, is not an easily diagnosable disorder or injury.

Loneliness is a subjective emotion so it is in a different category entirely. But just like that painful ankle can dictate your day – there's no chance you're following through on those promises to join a five-a-side team, after all – so too can emotions. If ignored, they can build up and cause physiological responses like a rise in the stress hormone cortisol. And simply seeking out more friends doesn't solve the problem. As I found, you can have many connections but if they're not deep or meaningful then you can still feel lonely. This is where running helped me mend the gap.

When I accepted the offer to run the London Marathon, a new world opened up before me. With every run, gym session or treadmill class came an invitation to join conversations within the running community. Rather than a half-arsed 'How are you?' running conversations start with, 'So you're running London, hey?' Now, this might not sound that revolutionary but it's the chance to chit-chat about a topic that you're both interested in. From the get-go you can connect and do a deep, conversational dive that feels like quality social contact. And, it doesn't just happen at races or run clubs. I've found that running has created new online conversations that have grown into offline relationships, too. It wasn't that long ago that I was rounding up a group of IG 'friends' to meet me on the start line of a half marathon.

Of course it would be irresponsible of me to say that running is a magical band-aid, and that as soon as you start your loneliness and your anxieties will heal. It's not and they won't. But I've definitely found it to be a useful outlet for emotions that can otherwise keep getting pumped around my body like a virus. When not using running as a way to meet and connect with others, I use this exercise like a vent on a pressure cooker.

In the past years (and chapters) I've been open and honest about my struggles with my London lifestyle; about the fact that, in the past, I've been so chronically stressed that I couldn't sleep, eat properly or respond to common situations in a rational manner. For many years, when things went haywire I didn't have a go-to coping mechanism. Sometimes I'd drink myself to blackout and pay for it the next day. Other times, I'd exercise myself into the ground. Neither one was an effective solution to make those tough days not seem as bad. In reality, they made them worse.

I'm not sure when the breakthrough happened, but in the past two years I have realised that my inbox or workload is, sadly, going nowhere. I've chosen a career in publishing, after all, and you don't need to be fully up to speed on *Media Week* to know that things are, er, challenging. Instead of wishing for a lighter workload I need to be better equipped to deal with what I'm dealt.

It started with lunchtime runs to put some temporary distance between myself and my job list. This then evolved into runs home to ensure that by the time I got through the door, I was able to switch off my work brain and enjoy two hours of relaxing before going to sleep and for it all to start again. I knew these well-planned runs made me feel better, but I wasn't really aware of how much they did until the summer of 2018.

That August, a former colleague and proper work pal lost his battle against depression. He became the third person I've known to take their own life. If the gut-wrenching and terribly sad fact that suicide is the *biggest* killer of young people in the UK hadn't hit home before, that summer it did. I found it really hard to process that the person who I'd shared jokes and some-times a terrible-tasting protein snack with was wrestling with his mental health and I hadn't known. He'd only recently emailed and asked to have lunch – was he going to let me in? – but I'd filed his email into my to-do list and, heartbreakingly, didn't deal with it before it was too late.

I found myself thinking about him and *that email* on my runs, especially when I ran past the crematorium where his funeral was held. My headspace would be filled with thoughts of him but also muddied by anger. Not necessarily at him but at myself: why did I not reply? Why had I not seen that all those days off sick with migraines were masking some-thing bigger? Why didn't I just make time for him? Often, I'd cry behind my running sunglasses or make myself sprint up the hill, using the gradient of the road to muffle the screams that so wanted to come out. Some days I'd just pause outside the doors of the crematorium and take five deep breaths before running on. It didn't really matter what happened on the run but the fact that something happened was key; running had become a cathartic release that helped me to not run away from my emotions, but actually deal with them.

The science of using running as a self-help mechanism has been well documented over the years: I mean, I'm far from the first one to say, 'Hey, running is good for your mental health,' but as the UK's mental-health crisis deepens, finding and encouraging any kind of solution is more important than ever before. Take journalist-turned-mental-health-advocate Bryony Gordon. Her book *Eat, Drink, Run* documents how, in her words, running saved her life.

'I remember running a half marathon when I was 53 days sober,' she told me. 'They let me out of rehab to do it. In fact,

I think running got me sober. It showed me that there was something different out there; a whole other world that I could be part of. It showed me how to respect my body.'

When Bryony was 12 years old she developed obsessive compulsive disorder (OCD), but back then, she didn't know what it was: 'No one was talking about mental illness back in the 90s and so I didn't know what was going on. I was scared and it snowballed. I developed really bad coping mechanisms to deal with it, like alcoholism, and my hair fell out because I was so stressed. And then I developed bulimia in a weird way to regain control again over my body.'

For years, Bryony abused her body with alcohol and drugs to silence the negative, irrational thoughts in her head. She shrugged off the notion that exercise was a better option because she wasn't a runner. But working in the mental-health space forced her to confront the issue head on: running really might help. So, wearing a pair of battered Converse, her husband's tracksuit bottoms and one of his Star Wars T-shirts, and using her daughter's Tommy Tippee cup as a water bottle, she set out on her first run. That run progressed into signing up for a marathon and ever since, she's been an open book on how running has improved her mental health.

She's not the only one. Since sharing her experience of coping with depression, Fearne Cotton regularly talks about her 'need to move' for good mental health. She'll go on a 5k just to give her overactive brain a break. And then there's Davina McCall, who runs for the sense of achievement, not the obvious fitness gains.

And so, it comes down to this. Running isn't a panacea for mental health but it can be your secret weapon in handling whatever life or your brain throws at you on any given day.

IN THE RUNNING FOR A MENTAL BOOST

That running is good for your physical health is
obvious, and you may well be familiar with (and fond
of) the mental buzz you get from it, too. But there's
more to it than that. The impact running can have,
both on your cognitive powers and your mental health,
is a burgeoning area of research. These are the
science-backed benefits worth chasing down.

Quicker thinking

If you're in need of an immediate mental pick-me-up,
and yet another coffee won't cut it, then it's best to
lace up your trainers. US researchers from the
University of Illinois[32] found that running can improve
your reasoning ability when answering complicated
questions, while separate science from National Taiwan
Sport University[33] suggests that half an hour of cardio
is enough to fire up your mental performance. And
what's best is that the benefits are instantaneous. If
you're flagging before an important meeting at work,
a 30-minute run is your speediest solution for faster
thinking.

High-performance brain power

Turn that one-off boost into a regular running habit
and you can double-down on the benefits. Beyond
keeping your grey matter on its toes, running can
actually trigger the growth of all-new brain tissue. It
drives neurogenesis and angiogenesis, which is the

growth of nerve cells and blood vessels that then combine to make your brain bigger. Until recently, it had been thought that you couldn't increase grey matter after childhood and that, after 20, the only route was decline. But research published in the journal PNAS[34] found that regular runners added 2 per cent to the size of their hippocampus and pumped up cognitive power, benefiting learning and memory. Further proof that heading to Parkrun every Saturday is the thinking person's decision.

Memory that goes the distance

And these benefits are no flash in the pan, either. In fact, they may well provide the ballast your brain needs against the march of time and ageing. As people live longer, the risk and incidence of dementia are, sadly, on the rise, but the long-term mental return of running may provide a level of protection. The *Lancet* found that physical inactivity is the strongest avoidable risk factor for dementia,[35] with other research[36] pinpointing regular time on the treadmill as a route to preventing cognitive decline. Every run is a step in the right direction for long-term brain health.

A kickstart to your mood

Beyond smarts in the office and at home, one of the biggest concerns today is mental health, and rightly so. Anxiety and depression are on the rise, and running can provide a fast-acting, free solution. For a quick uptick in mood, you'd do well to flood your system with some post-run endorphins. Studies have shown[37] the sweet spot for endorphin production is a comfortably hard effort (think the gruelling but very useful tempo runs discussed in chapter 3), while research at Oxford University found exercising in groups (chapter 2) could increase endorphin release, too.[38] Running also triggers your brain to release substances called endocannabinoids, which sounds a little like cannabis for a reason, as they promote feelings of calm. Challenging but not all-out efforts (70–85 per cent of maximum heart rate) are the key to unlocking this benefit from your brain's natural pharmacy.

And a route to crushing stress long term

Much like the long-term benefits to brain power of turning your time in trainers into a habit, regular running can help to keep a lid on anxiety and depression *ad infinitum*, too. A study published in the *Journal of Psychiatry & Neuroscience*[39] identified increased levels of the mood-elevating neurotransmitter serotonin in the brains of runners. The suggestion being that the more you run, the more happy hormones there are coursing through your brain, helping to keep your head above water in times of stress and sadness. It's a theory backed up by another study,[40] published in the *Journal of Sports Medicine and Physical Fitness*, which found that physical activity helped to lower patients' score on the Depression, Anxiety and Stress Scale (DASS).

'There is no such thing as failure, only feedback'

Follow The Leader

Andrew Cohen-Wray is an athlete with over two and a half decades of competitive experience who wants to help people of any sporting ability achieve the same mindset used by top-level athletes. His goal is simple: to offer the same service that Olympians receive to the everyday athlete. Thanks to his wealth of experience at the top levels of sport he's primed to do just that – I'll hand over to him to explain.

ON YOUR MARKS, MINDSET, GO!

The mindset you adopt drives everything. It is the root of your attitude, which then dictates your behaviour. All of this is created by your internal dialogue, and depending on whether that dialogue is positive or negative, it can drive you towards success or failure. It sounds hackneyed to suggest it's all in your head, but hold that thought . . .

Obviously, a negative mindset is going to be extremely limiting and that is precipitated by negative language in your internal dialogue – examples of which might sound painfully familiar. Phrases like, I can't, I shouldn't, I'm not good enough, all work against you to create a negative attitude. That attitude sounds like: I don't want to go for a run because . . . I'm not good enough, I'm not fast enough, my bum looks too big. Finally, that then drives your behaviours. You talk yourself out of going for a run, feel worse and so the negative mindset becomes self-perpetuating.

If this sounds familiar then take the initiative – you need to tune in to that negative dialogue and listen to what you're saying to yourself. And then analyse it. Ask yourself, 'Would I talk to my friend or partner like that?' If not, then why are you allowing yourself to talk to *you* like it?

You have to keep asking the why. Why am I acting like that? Why am I thinking like that? Why am I not driven right now? And once you get five 'whys' down the line you'll get closer to working it out. You could be down because you've eaten a load of crap today. So ask why you ate crap. Maybe you ate crap because you didn't prepare lunch. Why didn't you prepare lunch? Maybe you didn't prepare lunch because you got home late from work and you're just too stressed at work to concentrate on anything. All of a sudden, there's your root problem and you can start working out how to find a solution.

You also need to realise that missing a run is OK and that plans are designed as a guide. Wednesday of week 8 may say that you need to do a 14-mile run but, well, that might not work for you because little Jonny has got to go to ballet. And that's fine. The schedule is a guide, not the law. You need to have the confidence to tweak it, to make it work around you and not let the stress of sticking to it spark negative dialogue.

GET ON TARGET WITH GOAL SETTING

When I see people on social media saying they don't want to go out running, they hate it and they can't be bothered, a lot of that comes down to motivation. It's a common problem. What they need is a goal. The biggest motivator is having a goal and vision of what you want to achieve and, importantly, how you want to do it.

In my world there are two types of goal. You have an outcome goal and you have process goals. Your outcome goal could be a finisher's medal at the London Marathon. It could be time derived. It could be to get a PB. And then what you need to do is to put process goals in place to get there.

With athletes we have an Olympic cycle, which is four years. As soon as Rio finished in 2016 it was back to day 1 and setting goals like, 'I want to win a gold medal in 2020.' That's the outcome goal and we work back from there. How fast do I need to run to win, for example. Then, what do I need to do to get there?

My business partner is a paralympian who won a bronze medal, and he breaks it down brilliantly and simply. Look at what time would be needed to run a paralympic 800m. Let's says he needs to get to a 1.55m or quicker, but he was running 1.59. Basically he needs to take off 4 seconds over 800m. That's a good 30–40m of distance he needs to make up to get gold. It sounds daunting. However, he sat down with his coach, and they broke it down into a second a year. Which when you break it down further then means that you need to be able to get it down by around 0.1 of a second every month. All of a sudden, that becomes quite manageable.

And so, rather than freaking yourself out by giving yourself the goal of 3 hours to run a marathon when you're only running 4 hours, you can break that down over a year. Then you realise that you need to get 5 minutes quicker every month, and can formulate the process steps to get you there.

The most important thing with any kind of process is reviewing progress. You need to do it constantly. It needs to be ingrained into your mindset. It's the difference between realising that you're not on target on day 1 week 2, not day 7 week 5. Equally, it can also help with the problem of knowing that you're doing enough. Review works both ways. It stops things from going badly, but it also backs things up when it is going well, to provide positive feedback and a boost to your confidence.

BOUNCING BACK FROM DEFEAT

Your running career will be plagued by both macro and micro defeats, ranging from long-term injury to a missed run. But I have a good saying that I share with my athletes – there's no such thing as failure, only feedback.

Think of it like a long-jump run-up. You put a marker down and you run down, put your foot on the board, jump and land in the sand. It's really simple. But if when you hit the board you get a no jump, you are given a number of how far you've gone over – 7cm, say. The way we look at it is not that you've failed but that you've jumped great and were 7cm over. That's your feedback. Adjust your run-up by 7cm, do it again and you'll nail it.

With running you can look at your own feedback. What went wrong? Were you running in the wrong heart-rate zone? Did you go out too fast? The trick is not to dwell on it, to draw a line in the sand and work out how to make it better. There are always solutions.

If what went wrong was that you ran out of steam on a hill, then the problem is that you lack strength. That can be fixed by tweaking your plan in the weights room. If you get a stitch, look at your diet. If you pulled something, is there a weakness or imbalance that you can even out? The biggest and best tip is always: listen to your body.

One of the best people I've worked with is Dai Green, who was a 400m runner and finished 4th at the Olympics. You may think that there is no worse place to finish in a race at that level. But when I spoke to him, he disagreed. He'd had a world of injury problems in the run-up to the games and only got the green light to run again in the February before having to compete in July. He did everything possible in the time and went into the race in the best shape he could. He missed out on gold by 0.3 seconds, but he didn't view it as a disappoint-ment. If he'd had another month could he have got that 0.3s? Possibly. But he didn't have another month, so tough shit – and he understood that.

You need to focus on yourself, rather than what's going on around you. Coming up short in a competition doesn't mean a failure on your part. There are so many things out of your control that get in the way. So you need to swap the focus from the result to how you feel you did. And if you did your best then that's a victory. The rest is all feedback that will only serve to help you get better in the future.

OUTRUNNING BOREDOM

I admit, running can be mind-numbing sometimes. Not every minute around the local park is a wonderful opportunity to clear your head. Sometimes it's a slog. The key is to tune in to your different senses and work out the most effective distrac-tion for you.

People often rely on running with music. If you're more of an auditory person that'll work. The music in your ears will overrule and drown out the negative dialogue. It switches off the other noise telling you to stop.

The other option is if you are a visual person. In this instance your preferred distraction is what you can see and so you need to pick runs that are interesting to look at. You need to give treadmills a very wide berth, and find new runs or run old loops in the opposite direction.

It's a weird truth that there's a problem with running the same routes on training runs beyond boredom, too. It's a psycho-logical thing. If you run a 10-mile training run and you get a stitch at mile 5, then you go and do the same loop again there's a high chance you'll get the same stitch around mile 5 again. It becomes a muscle memory of 'I always struggle around 5 miles'. You end up persuading yourself it's going to happen and it does.

Consistency is key for race practice because you can test progress, but on your long runs, then variety is a necessity. If you run the same routes you'll have the same problems.

HOW TO BREAK THROUGH THE WALL

This may come as consolation or frustration to anyone who's come clattering into the metaphorical wall and been forced to pull out of a race, but it has nothing to do with mental strength. The wall is a glycogen depletion – you've simply run out of energy. It's a nutrition issue and not a mindset issue. It's good news therefore that it wasn't your resolve that gave up (you're likely tougher than you think), but frustrating in that an extra, well-timed energy gel could well have powered you across the finish line.

However, that's not to say that running isn't tough and having the perseverance to push on can be learned. In my opinion, if you are training for a half marathon or a marathon then you should be doing all the dark stuff in training. People say that in races they go to a really dark place, but actually racing should be the easy bit – the icing on the cake.

This may present a slightly different perspective from your normal running plans – further proof that there are plenty of ways to skin a cat and that the onus is on the individual to work out what's most effective for them – but I'll programme runs that are 28, 30, 32 miles for my athletes. Most plans won't take you above 20. However, if you only do 20 miles and on race day you have to run 26, then you've got 6 miles that you've never done before. What you're doing then is you're creating stress, anxiety and taking yourself out of your comfort zone. From a mentality standpoint, you may well start to lose confidence as a result. Confidence is your belief in your ability to perform a task well, based on a previous experience. The key to confidence is past experience.

I realise that I'm not talking with pro runners here, and if you're building up as a beginner over a 16-week marathon plan, then you don't have time to work in 30-mile runs. But if you're new to running and working up to your first 10k race, then absolutely it will help you to go out in training and run 12k. Come the start line you'll be full of confidence because you'll know what to expect. You've got it in the bag.

On The Run With . . . Charlie Martin

Charlie Martin is a game changer in motorsport. She has fought continuously to overcome adversity throughout her life, from having lost both her parents at a young age to realising she identified as transgender, transitioning to live as female midway through her career in 2012. Throughout this, running has acted as a salve, helped her to work through adversity and become stronger. This is her story.

AL: There have been some incredible highs and lows during your journey, and you're certainly riding high now, but can you take me back to explain what it was like growing up?

CM: Of course. It was really confusing on a number of levels. Firstly, coming to the realisation that I felt like I was in the wrong body and the wrong gender. And then on top of that I didn't really have any reference point for what trans was. There was no internet and trans people weren't visible. You didn't see any trans people in jobs or with careers.

And so from that I started worrying about this compromise, thinking that if I want to be who I am, then I'm going to have to massively downgrade my aspirations of what I want to achieve. Fundamentally, I felt that society was going to view me as this weird person who doesn't conform to norms and so I'd have to live on the fringes as an outcast.

The only trans people you saw were on film and they were only portrayed in a negative way, or as some kind of joke element. There was nothing positive about being trans as far as I could see, apart from being who you wanted to be.

Beyond that I was also confused because I grew up wanting to be a fighter pilot. I wanted to do all the typical activities that young boys were into. I didn't have sisters growing up; I grew up on *Star Wars*, *GI Joe* and *Top Gun*. Back then, and even now, everything I could see or read relating to trans people protrayed this ideal of a trans female having to be overtly feminine, attracted to someone of the opposite sex and growing up wanting to wear pink. Which wasn't me.

AL: And so did gender stereotyping, even in the trans community, make everything more difficult?

CM: Yes, there was a massive disconnect. By and large the majority of my interests were what many people would refer to as typically male.

At the time I felt like I didn't fit in because I didn't even fit into the norm of being trans. I felt like even if I came out to trans people that I wouldn't fit in with them. Everything told me that I needed to be super-feminine. And that's not to say I didn't want to wear dresses, but I also wanted to be my own version of me, and it's why I'm so passionate about breaking down gender stereotypes today.

For me, that was a massive barrier between becoming the person that I needed to be. It was only later in life when I felt more confident about myself that I thought people can take me as they find me, but it's not that easy when you're 10!

AL: And to a 10-year-old the concept of mental health doesn't even exist. The idea of being anxious or being depressed. And so, when you're feeling those emotions, I imagine it makes it all the more confusing?

CM: Yes, absolutely. When you don't have people to talk to and to share your thoughts with and don't know how to articulate those feelings, the easiest and most common response is just to keep it bottled up.

AL: How did these feelings then progress from childhood into your teens? Teeanage years are tough at the best of times!

CM: I'll be honest, it was a real mess. I did try and throw myself into things and try to keep myself busy, but I also discovered alcohol quite young and that was a major coping mechanism. I had bouts of depression, anxiety and anorexia. I just felt like I was being pulled in two directions the whole time. Because on the one hand I wanted to transition. And though there wasn't any particular moment, I'd known that's what I wanted to be from when I was 10 or 11. I'd already spoken to my mum about it and a load of school friends.

But my dad had just died from cancer and I was really struggling. I was torn because, as I've mentioned, I thought that transitioning would mean compromising. Bear with me because this sounds a little complicated, but I really thought I was going to have to give up what made me me to become this other version of me that I wanted to be . . .

AL: I can certainly see how that would get confusing!

CM: And so I felt like I had to choose. On the one hand I wanted to hold on to who I was, but on the other hand, I wanted to change. I wanted to change my body – which was a major part of where my eating disorder came from – because I wanted to look androgynous. Being thin and growing my hair helped to offset the fact that my voice was breaking and that I was having to deal with body hair.

The testosterone as I went through puberty was messing with my head, as it does for all teens, and although I'd given up on my dreams of being a fighter pilot because I was terrible at physics and maths, I then set my sights on joining the Marine Commandos. I wanted to push myself and do something that was completely at odds with transitioning.

I thought, if I can't have that, then I'm going to do this one thing that takes me so far away from transitioning that I have no time to think about it. It's a common thing and I've met trans women who joined the Marines. Their mindset was, if I can't have that then sod it, I'm going to do the most out-there thing that will totally remove me from that space, so it's not going to even be an option.

It's a yin and yang. I'd have periods of being settled on one outcome and then I'd switch back.

AL: And so from wanting to be in the Marines, how did motorsport come into your life?

CM: One of my friends at school, his dad raced and we would go away at weekends together and go racing. And then when we started getting our first cars as friends, *Max Power* magazine was a thing, and so car culture was always part of my life growing up. Then that same friend started to race as a natural progression from his dad, so I looked at him and thought, that's something I'd like to do and something I thought I could do.

The year I left university I was 23 and I bought a car for a few hundred quid. I needed to build it up from scratch. But I'm the kind of person who, once I've decided to do something, I just go for it. And when people didn't think I could do it, it just made me more determined to prove them wrong. And I started racing the next year.

AL: Racing is a traditionally masculine arena to be in. Was that a struggle?

CM: No, because that's the life I was living then. I was in a relationship with a woman who I then ended up getting married to. And outwardly I didn't identify as trans. I was, for all intents and purposes *'just a regular guy'*. And I'd never had girlfriends until that point – it was the first time that I'd fallen in love. It felt right and being with that person was the most amazing thing to ever happen, so all of a sudden being trans was no longer important to me. I was so happy. And so at that time I felt pretty secure in the version of the person I was portraying. For five years, everything was perfect. I was in love. I bought a house. I was racing.

But things in my life tend to move in cycles of everything seeming OK and, as a result, me burying everything that doesn't fit with that ideal. It then bubbles away under the surface until it eventually reappears.

I'd been having counselling during this time and working out ways of dealing with how I felt in the hope that I could stay in this perfect life that I had created for myself. Because I didn't want that to end, but at the same time I was really struggling. The problem was I couldn't do both things, and that was causing a lot of inner turmoil, which really came to a head at the end of 2011.

I had a nervous breakdown and was suicidal. And that's simply because I couldn't see a way out. I essentially had two options. One was to stay with my partner for ever and be really happy with her, but then also deal with this hidden part of my life, that at that time was unbearable. The other option was to leave behind that partner who meant so much to me, with no guarantee of what transitioning was going to be like. It was a leap of faith into the unknown. And so the way to not have to make that decision was to take my life.

AL: Thankfully you did eventually make a positive decision. So what was the defining factor?

CM: It was a combination of things. I realised suicide wasn't the solution and that it would only cause a lot of pain for everyone around me. I lost both of my parents to cancer early in my life and so I felt an obligation to them. They wouldn't have wanted me to do it, but what they would want was for me to be the person I needed to be. And so transitioning became the only way forward.

AL: Was this another example of when you set your mind to something, you go all out?

CM: Yes, once I'd made that decision I went at it all guns blazing. Once I'd made the decision I felt free, and there was no pressure. I finally knew I was doing the right thing.

AL: And what has it been like for your mental health since then?

CM: There was probably a period of six months talking to friends and family where it would be awkward and anxious, but after that it became easy. I remember the first time I told one of my close friends about how I had been struggling my whole life and that it was difficult to explain, but I felt I needed to change and that I was trans. And all they said was, what are you worrying about, that's fine, that's amazing and I'm still your friend.

And that all boils down to what I had built up in my own mind. I had turned it into this awful thing that no one was going to understand. And many do the same and that's why so many people end up spending a lifetime bottling these things up and not talking about them. You build it into this monstrous thing and all perspective is lost.

AL: And did being honest and the support of those around you help you to make sense of the fear and break it down?

CM: Yes. And one of the other major things that helped me was people on YouTube. I hadn't seen real trans people before in a way that I could connect with. I saw that they had normal lives and saw how they changed as people they grew into their new selves. It was a very powerful thing that made it seem more possible.

AL: And I know that running was a major part in helping you to deal with these emotions, too.

CM: Absolutely. When I was at school, running was my most hated thing. But equally I was never sporty, either. And when I left university I realised that I'd had a long period of drinking way too much and doing no exercise. However, I had no sport or hobby that I could do that I could use to get moving, and so running became the obvious thing. It's simple. It's the one thing that really everyone can do – you just need to do it.

And so without any real ambition I just started running a bit. I found it really hard, but I persevered. And then after a year a couple of friends got in touch to say they were running a half marathon – and I'm quite competitive – I thought maybe I should give it a go. I started getting a bit more serious and built myself up to do a race with them. And the first time I did it I remember so clearly being really impressed and proud of myself for the time I achieved.

It wasn't fast but it was the first time in my life that I felt a sense of pride and self-belief like that. I'd played rugby badly at school, but with running there was no team to rely on – it was just me. And so I wanted to build on that feeling.

Then in that dark period at the end of 2011 I was running a lot. It was a real release for me. When you've got a lot of stress and shit going around in your life, when you go for a run, I find that your body gets into this natural rhythm. I don't focus on my problems so much. I just sort through things in my mind automatically and things just seem to fall into their natural place. It's almost like the subconscious mind takes over and starts to work through things for you.

AL: Have you had any eureka moments while running that have been crucial to your mental health?

CM: I remember when I'd made the decision to transition in the beginning of 2012. I remember running and thinking for the first time in my life that I was running towards something, rather than running away. At that time I had started living on my own after living with my now ex for eight years. I used to come home every day and there would be a deathly silence. I found it really hard to come home to. But running was my antidote, I would put my trainers on and then I would just run.

AL: And was that because you knew it would help your mental strength?

CM: Subconsciously, yes, I think so. Because I knew that once I'd done it, I would get home, feel great and be in a completely different frame of mind. And then also because I was running so much I was also getting really, really fit. I was running 6-minute miles and really enjoying it, and that then compounded how I felt mentally. For the first time I felt in control of my body and my body was doing these amazing things that I could be proud of. It really transformed my mental state. If I hadn't been running at that point in my life the future could have turned out very differently for me. It really was a game changer.

AL: And so finally, what kind of message of advice would you give to people going through something similar, either as someone transitioning or struggling with their mental health?

CM: I think that, beyond the advice that you see most places today, the individual piece of advice that I can give would be to look to YouTube. It really helped me to get to know and feel comfortable in the trans community. Without realising it, I spent my entire life with only cisgender friends, but on YouTube and then meeting in person through YouTube, I was able to talk to people who could relate to what I was going through. And that same principle extends to people who are suffering from anxiety and depression, because those accounts, people and communities exist there, too. You can talk to people who relate to what you're experiencing, and that will be such a wonderful help.

Your Chapter 9 Action Plan

- Every time you hit a stumbling block, ask yourself why until you find the root cause, and then set about finding a solution

- Set end goals and process goals that will give you the motivation to keep moving forward even when the going gets tough

- Review, review, review your progress to ensure you're going in the right direction and to give yourself the opportunity for self-congratulation

- Work out if you're an auditory or visual person to beat running boredom

- Do the hard parts in training to build up confidence. Confidence comes from experience

CHAPTER 10

See You At The Start Line

My Journey

On any running journey you're likely to come a hell of a long way, both physically and mentally. And that journey never ends, but over the past few years I've found that races serve as an excellent way for me to check in with my progress as well as give me the motivation to keep moving and improving. They're sometimes scary but always worth more than the weight of the gold hanging-round your neck come the finish line.

Rarely have I felt fully prepared on the eve of a race. Flashes of missed runs and skipped recovery protocols too often haunt my thoughts. And if I'm not stewing over a less-than-perfect training cycle then I'm mentally counting down the hours until I need to get up and prepare because, of course, I didn't sort out my race-day essentials until the very last minute. No matter how many times I sign up, the state of 'maranoia' I work myself into is real.

I've always wanted to be the person who preps their kit bag

the weekend before a race, so when the 24-hour countdown begins I have to give it nothing more than a cursory glance. My evening would then be free for chowing down on carbs, and reading in the bath with a lavender-scented candle and a face mask. And perhaps, if I was really going for it, a 10-minute visualisation of race day. There would be no screens, no mad Googling of 'how to get to the red start pen' and definitely no endless attempts at the perfect flat lay. That shit would've been done days ago, I would just add my filter and send it to the Instagram grid. Job done. But sadly, it's never been the case. I've always been someone who procrastinates until the 11th hour, and race day always arrives at 6am should I be well-rested and ready . . . or not.

I distinctly remember one Saturday evening before a race. After last-minute swotting up on London Marathon tips, I was full of regret about not ordering a personalised race vest. How on earth was I going to make it around the course without spectators' cries of 'keep going *Amy*' and 'you're doing great *Amy*'? My race-day anxiety told me that, in fact, I wouldn't, so I decided to fashion a name tag out of card, a black Sharpie and a stencil to pin onto my race shirt. I stayed up far too late doing this. Had I worn a sleep tracker that night I'm sure it would have graded my sleep worse than my attempt at an A-level in politics. For the record, the results for that particular test came back 'ungraded'. But unlike this academic failing, in running I've always tried to learn from my mistakes.

Take the DIY name tag; I've never done that again. My one and only attempt didn't survive the race. In fact, my sweat caused the black marker pen to run onto my skin and down my legs before the whole thing disintegrated. I ended up with what looked liked pretty severe varicose veins and bits of card all over me.

Another disaster that springs to mind is the year that I didn't really grasp the idea of 'carb loading'. Rather than prioritise eating pasta, grains and bread to build up my energy stores, I simply ate more of *everything*. I filled my boots and went to bed stuffed. The next morning I woke up and yes, my boots were full but so were my bowels – not great when you haven't budgeted enough time for multiple toilet visits before leaving the house. I ended up queueing for the portaloo in the race village and, of course, there was no toilet paper. I was forced to use the inside of a toilet roll as makeshift tissue, both painful and not that efficient. I'm sure I'm not the first one to have done this; however, if one takeaway sticks with you from this book make it this: always pack a safety tissue in your start-line bag. Tuck it in your bra or stuff it in your bumbag, just keep it close until you set off.

My list of 'if I only I had' could go on and on, but I'll share just one more from the Richmond Half Marathon – a race that I ran with my sister, Emma. At school, Emma was always an athletic person; she wiped the floor with me at track, field *and* in the swimming pool. While I didn't really progress past my 100m badge and had to learn front crawl at the age of 28, my sister had sports badge after sports badge to adorn her school swimming cossies. But after 18, while I dabbled in different training, my sister's interest in organised movement fizzled out. So when she asked me if I wanted to run a half marathon, I was surprised. At different ages and paces, we'd never planned to run it together, however, I wasn't quite prepared for what was to follow. For the first mile or so, I tried to trail behind Emma and her friend, eager to run as a group. Sister solidarity and all that. But, it was painful. I wasn't used to running at their pace and I also felt like a weird stalker running just behind them. I didn't want to offend them by running on (my sister's friend has a disability) but was also aware that trailing them like traffic on the M25 was probably stressing them out, too. So, I asked Em if she would mind if I ran on; she didn't, so off I went. But I hadn't loaded up my phone with an offline playlist and much of this race is on a towpath with patchy signal. My only option was to play the three songs I had downloaded onto my phone, which was an excruciating mix of Justin Bieber, Celine Dion and a chanting yoga song. It sent me round the bend.

I got through the next 11(ish) miles on sheer determination to finish. I was elated when I did because as beautiful as the long stretches of river paths are, Richmond isn't a big race, or at least it wasn't at the time. When I ran it there weren't many water stations to break up the course, nor were there many supporters to cheer us runner folk on. And, as it wasn't a closed course, at times you had to deal with non-runners trying to go about their normal Sunday. Like one man and his labradoodle, which decided to run after me barking until I gave in and allowed it to have the rest of my banana. Of course, he then just sniffed it before running off.

When I made it to the finish I was ready for creature comforts only to realise that my warm clothes were locked in my sister's car. They wouldn't be that much longer than me, would they? Ten minutes went by. Then 15, then 30. I stood shivering in my sweat-soaked and now rain-sodden kit at the finish line. I kept bouncing around like a *Riverdance* reject to keep warm, but it was a losing battle. I have inherited Raynaud's syndrome from my mother so as soon as the mercury drops below 10 degrees I start to lose blood in my fingers and morph into the colour of a ghoul. I was also starting to worry: where was Em? By now, the finishers were getting few and far between; the medics were treating the injured who'd been rescued from the course and Em's friend had crossed the finish line after saying they'd split up around 8 miles.

As the race was too small to have a sweeper bus to pick up runners going too slowly to finish, I decided to track back. After 10 minutes, I found my sister shuffling along like a

95-year-old man. What didn't help matters was that she'd managed to tangle her neck in her headphone wires so she was also trudging along with her head cocked to one side. All her will to either pick up her feet or engage any muscle group had gone. This was now an exercise in mind over matter to make it to the end. I put aside all thoughts of numb fingers and toes to be there by her side as she crossed the line.

Later that evening, while using a red wine bottle as a foam roller (a terrible idea that made sense only having drained the contents of said bottle) we reviewed the catalogue of errors of the race: it was foolhardy to think we'd be the same pace after not doing *any* runs together; it was unorganised to not have loaded 'offline music' onto our pods, and not using the bag drop was a terrible idea. I'd risked hypothermia; my sister had experienced unnecessary pain by running a race without proper training or kit.

In the beginning, obstacles like those I've shared can trip us up, but as time goes on, you realise that while you might stumble at the time, you won't stay down for long. It's these moments of discomfort, the ones that you are forced to face head on, that can cause you to ask 'why?' and 'what's the point?' and sometimes weep behind your sunglasses, that ultimately increase your resilience and help you to become the best runner you can be.

After Eliud Kipchoge broke the 2-hour marathon barrier, he told the breathless press: 'I'm sending a message to every individual in this world that when you work hard, when you actually concentrate, when you set your priorities high, when you actually set your goals, and put them in your heart and in your mind, you will accomplish, without any question.' And he's right. You will accomplish your goal, it's just you who gets to decide how much discomfort you'll put yourself through on the day to get there. Whatever you're working towards, be it 5k or the London Marathon, you can do it. In the words of Mo Farah: 'Don't dream of winning, train for it!'

'There is a time and pace for everyone'

Follow The Leader

Since her first marathon in 2013 Camilla Langlands has run more than 148 marathons. That's over 20 a year. By the time you read this, she'll have run many more, and many as a pacer. Here she joins me to detail her plan, designed to help you make the most of every minute.

OVERCOMING NERVES

It's difficult: you need to think of the marathon, or a half marathon, as just like any of your long training runs, because in terms of distance, it is.

The temptation is to think of race day as a completely different phenomenon, and that's part of the allure, it's what makes it exciting. But when that excitement spills over into anxiety it will pay to remember that, realistically, it's only going to be slightly longer than one of your Sunday-run-days, and the cheers of the crowd can push you through that, no problem.

I like to think of race day as the glory lap. It's a celebration of all the hard work you've done up until you hit the start line. That way you still get to treat it as an occasion in your head, but also realise that, in many ways, you've been here before and, most importantly, you've got this.

PACKING YOUR BAG

Before most races you're given a clear bag to fill with whatever you want, which you hand in at the start and are given back at the end. Be mindful that because it's so busy at the finish it may take a while to find family and friends, so, in addition to your winner's goodie bag, this is your post-race self-care package. Pack accordingly.

Start with a change of clothes. You may be lucky and the sun will be out. But then again, it's Britain. Once you cross the finish line you'll cool down very quickly and your sweat-soaked kit will get cold. A comfy pair of leggings and sweatshirt will work wonders. A pair of sliders is wonderful, too. Even experienced runners can finish 26.2 with blisters, and unlacing your tired feet will undoubtedly result in a sigh of relief.

Other than that, some baby wipes and a hairbrush will make all the difference when it comes to your victory photographs. Oh, and a sandwich. Always pack a sandwich. Yes, your family might be taking you out for a well-deserved celebratory meal, but nothing will compare to that first bite of carbs. Running a race is hungry work, you know.

FIND A PEN PAL

You'll be surprised at just how many people are at the starting line at races and you'd be forgiven for finding it daunting. But most of all, it can slow things down and you'll be in the pen for well over 30 minutes, which is a long time to mull over the reality of the next few hours. If you get nervous, find a pacer and say hello. We'll have big flags on our backs and will be easy to spot. Usually we become a bit of a hotspot for people to gather around and if you say hello to us you'll also say hello to lots of other runners all in the same boat. It's a nice opportunity to make friends and hear other people's stories but also just to take your mind off of the run and pass the time.

LAST MEAL

It's an early start. If you're smart, you'll have loaded up with food the night before and got out of bed in time to have a decent breakfast. However, the journey to the start line and the waiting in the pen will take time, so keep a banana or a cereal bar handy. If you're the type of person who relies on running gels to fuel during the race, then putting some real food in your tummy before the race can make you feel much better.

INVEST IN GPS

For me, having a GPS sports watch is invaluable. You can set them up to do pretty much anything, except run the race for you. At its most simple, it works out what pace you're running, which you can then match to your target times. Or, if you want the watch to work out that target for you, some can – for example, if you want to cross the line in under five hours in a marathon then it'll advise you to run between 11- and 11:30-minute miles.

DON'T PANIC IF YOU START FAST

That said, the pacers do often pace the first half of a race a minute or two faster, which allows for a very gradual fade in the second half. But they're doing that with quite a lot of experience and they're building it in gradually over the course miles. If you are running with the pacer and you think that they're running a little bit faster in the first half, that's probably the case, so don't be alarmed. They definitely know what they're doing. Stick with them and I guarantee they'll get you to the end in good time.

TALK TO THE PACERS

Making people feel comfortable and relaxed is an important role for us as pacers. It can get busy around us, and I wouldn't advocate elbowing others out the way to come and have a chinwag, but if you're next to us and want to talk, please do. Chatting, especially in the early stages, can be a great way to ease some of the nerves and anxieties. However, that chatter does have a habit of dying out after around an hour for obvious reasons . . .

WATCH OUT FOR WATER

The first thing I would say about the hydration stations is to be careful. It sounds dramatic, but there are bottles everywhere. Unfortunately, because they distribute bottles that are quite big and people don't drink that much fluid at a time, a lot of the bottles are left on the floor half-full. They're easy to trip up on. I've seen it happen. And that would be such a disappointing way for your race to end.

HYDRATION TAKES TIME

Taking on water at full speed isn't easy, especially among the throngs of other racers trying to get a drink. I would recommend slowing down and walking while you grab a drink – although this will take a bit of practice in your training; just to be sure you can get going again! But it's a good time to collect your thoughts and make sure you're taking on enough water. However, even if it only takes place over 10 metres, it'll slow you down, so be mindful of that. When you take a look at your next split, you might be 30 seconds down. Don't panic and try to make that up in the next mile. Be brave and stick to your pace and claw it back 5 seconds at a time. Slow and steady will always win.

ASSUME YOU'RE GOING TO RUN FURTHER

I'm sorry to be the bearer of bad news, but the roads in races are so wide and so busy that all the weaving from side to side means you'll likely have to go further than 10k, 13.1 or 26.2 to cross the line and in some cases that can add on another few minutes, which can be disheartening when you think you're edging closer to the end. Don't let it. Think of it as added value as this last stretch is always surrounded by crowds and they'll cheer you on.

'THIS TOO SHALL PASS'

This is a quote from my mum and she uses it with me in everyday life, but also in running. If you're really struggling or you're hitting up against the wall, just remember that the feeling will pass (and hopefully that will be before the race ends, too!). I find that if you stay calm, work with it and remember it's only temporary then you'll pick up again. Never let it get you down; the aim in every run is to enjoy every single minute of it that you can.

On The Run With . . . Kathrine Switzer

In 1967 Kathrine Switzer broke new ground for runners like you and me by becoming the first female to officially run a marathon. For the past 50 years she has gone on to pioneer for progress and helped to empower women around the world through running. Consider her the OG of #fitspo.

AL: You've been a cult hero for a long time, but I've heard that there are some misconceptions flying around the internet . . .

KS: Everyone says that I was the first woman to run the Boston Marathon when actually I was the first one to officially *register* and run. Roberta Louise 'Bobbi' Gibb jumped out of the bushes and ran the year before but as she didn't have a bib number, there wasn't the controversy or coverage.

AL: Was Bobbi your inspiration to sign up?

KS: The inspiration for my doing it was my coach, Arnie. He was the university mailman and was training with the Syracuse cross-country team where I was a student. And he had run the Boston Marathon 15 times. I told him that I wanted to run it, and then he let me know the only problem there is that women aren't allowed to run. I said, 'What do you mean?' He said that women can't run 26.2 because they are too weak and too fragile. I was furious. We argued and I told him about the story from the previous year and he said, 'If *any* woman could do it, you could, but you would have to prove it to me. If you ran the distance in practice, I'd be the first to take you to Boston.'

But Arnie was really worried that he was going to be blamed if I did run it and it ruined my legs or, worst of all, stopped me from having children. His biggest fear was that running that far would somehow reduce your reproductive capability. He stuck to his word, though. We did a 31-mile practice run together and he then helped me to sign up to the race.

AL: Why do you think he said you were fragile even though he was coaching you through intense training sessions as part of your cross-country fitness plan?

KS: He thought all women were fragile. That's what everyone thought. And women themselves still do; they view themselves as the weaker sex. The interesting thing there is that the more research we do the more we find out that women have more endurance and stamina than men. We don't have the speed, the power or the strength – but if you want to go for ever then that's where women come to the fore. The future is really very exciting for women. We're outperforming men.

AL: How did you view yourself at the time?

KS: I thought that the whole thing was just a joke. Obviously I felt weaker than men – my older brother was faster, stronger and bigger than me. But that's just puberty kicking in. The hormones. I never felt fragile. I definitely knew at 15 that I was the fastest of the girls but wasn't as fast as the guys. And also I think it is important to say that I never felt fragile, but I loved being feminine. I didn't mind sweating and working out, but I also loved lipstick and sexy underwear.

AL: Did you ever worry about any of the comments? Was there any doubt in your mind about women being able to run long distances?

KS: It wasn't even a thought. Running was intoxicating to me. The more I ran the more powerful I felt. And the more you run the more you feel you can handle. If I ever got tired or bombed during a race I knew that it was because of poor pacing or poor nutrition, I never had a sense of fear about it.

AL: Let's talk about the lead-up to your momentous day in 1967. How did you enter the race if it was for men only?

KS: First, there were no rules written saying it was a men-only race. Next, there was nothing about gender on the entry form. Third, my coach told me it was OK for me to enter and in fact I must enter the race properly for my run to count. Lastly, I signed my name with my initials, K. V. Switzer. So the officials probably thought K stood for a man's name.

AL: Why do you sign your name with your initials?

KS: Because my name Kathrine was mis-spelled on my birth certificate and around age 12 I got tired of it being mis-spelled all the time. (You see, there is no 'e' in the middle of my name; normally it is spelled Katherine.) I also wanted to be a writer and admired authors like J. D. Salinger and E. E. Cummings, so I thought using my initials was a cool, writer-ly kind of thing to do.

AL: How long did you give yourself to get race ready?

KS: I remember it was after new year that we had the argument and Arnie subsequently agreed to take me. So we trained from 10 January to 19 April, which was the date of the marathon. And we did the 31-mile trial run about 10 days before that. It wasn't much recovery time, but we didn't think as much about that back then. The thing I do remember is that all the blisters and lacerations on my feet from running that trial still hadn't healed by the time I got to Boston. Before that three-month period, we'd never run more than 10 miles (we used to run 6 miles every day and then at the weekend we would ramp it up to 10). But for Boston we jumped from 18 to 26, but 26 actually turned into 31.

AL: Did you tell your friends you were training for Boston?

KS: The night after the 31-miler I told my boyfriend. He and my coach then blabbed it to the head coach. I found out later that they had a bet, a bottle of whisky, on whether I could actually do it.

AL: I heard your boyfriend also had some pretty contentious opinions at the time too . . .

KS: Yes! He was a hammer thrower at the time, training to become an Olympian. He was a brilliant athlete but he was a big guy. He said if you can do it then I can do it. I argued, no no, it's 26 miles and I've trained for it. He said it didn't matter, if I could do it, he could. So we went to run it together.

He did come in handy though because he was actually the guy who punched the race official when they were trying to take me off the course in the famous picture. Even better, however, was around the halfway mark when he really had to slow down and and started walking. He tried to make me slow down with him but I wouldn't and I ended up beating him by an hour and a half.

AL: At what point in the race did the official attack you?

KS: At about the 1½-mile mark, so I still had over 24 miles to run.

AL: When Jock the race manager tried to force you off the course, what were you feeling?

KS: I was scared to death. I just wanted to get away from him and I couldn't because he wouldn't let go. I was very, very scared because he was out of control, he was attacking me. My coach was trying to get him off and that's when it came to my boyfriend having to punch him to the ground. My inclination between fight or flight has always been flight. I was humiliated, of course, but then I became determined.

AL: There are famous photos of this incident. How did they take those photos?

KS: The photo truck was right in front of us and the press and officials' bus was alongside of us, working their way from the back of the race pack to the front. The official jumped off the bus and attacked me . . . right in full view of the photographers taking pictures from the back of the truck. It was very bad timing for the official, but it was very good timing for women's rights. The photo of the incident was flashed around the world and is now in Time-Life's book, *100 Photos that Changed the World.*

AL: You said that this happened early on in the race. How were you able to refocus?

KS: It was really hard because all the adrenaline had drained out of all of us. It wasn't just me, it was my trainer too. But about 10k later our energy came back and we got back into it . . . until the 22-mile mark when it started to get hard again, as it always does. But there was no way that I wasn't going to finish. I told my coach I'm going to do it on my hands and my knees if I have to, and I would have. But then when I crossed the line I actually felt great. My energy came back once again and I was really, really proud of myself.

Although, to be honest, crossing the end was actually a little anticlimactic. We'd had all this trauma at the beginning and mixed response from the crowd. And then towards the end, my coach, who hadn't run the race in about three years, didn't recognise the end. He didn't realise that it had been changed – he thought that we were being deliberately misdirected so that we didn't finish. It turns out that we weren't but it's interesting that that was a thought because, for my book, I went through old newspaper clippings and found one that said the [race] officials had approached the police – who were diverting traffic and guiding runners – to pull me from the race. Thankfully, the police refused.

AL: Did you get in trouble for running the Boston Marathon?

KS: Yes, the official who attacked me had me disqualified from the race and then expelled from the Amateur Athletic Union, the sport's governing body, for a whole list of reasons, one of which was running with men. Plus, there were a lot of negative press reports and plenty of hate mail.

AL: Were you interviewed at the finish line?

KS: Yes, but we had to get our guard back up again because the journalists were so unkind to me. One guy said, 'You're never going to run again are you, this is a joke?' Another asked, 'What are you trying to prove – can't you just give men their own thing?' I got pretty snippy. I said, 'I'm not trying to prove anything, I'm here to run and the marathon is never a joke. And as for never running, well you're going to read a news story in the future about a little old lady of 85 who died in Central Park doing a training run. That'll be me.' I gave as good as I got.

AL: Did the official ever apologise?

KS: Not really, but he did give me a kiss six years later on the starting line of the 1973 Boston Marathon and we eventually became good friends.

AL: How has the Boston Marathon experience changed your life?

KS: In just about every way because by the time I finished the race, I was inspired to become a better athlete myself and create opportunities for other women in running. All this led to several interesting careers, almost all of which I designed for myself and are connected to running and social change. The 1967 Boston Marathon also told me I could persevere over anything. And it has helped me to be pretty fearless in other ways, too.

AL: How does it feel to know that we're creeping towards it being a 50/50 split in that race?

KS: Yes, it's great. At some races they are now up at 70 per cent women. There are more women competing in races in the

US and Canada than there are men. But despite progress here and in Western Europe there are still problems in South America and in the Middle East where women are being culturally restricted. I've spent the last 52 years working towards giving women equality and setting up races all over the world that allow women to compete, and then getting women's marathon into the Olympic Games – that to me was the crowning achievement of my career.

AL: Why was it so important to get the women's marathon into the Olympic Games?

KS: Because I knew when the world saw women in the most difficult of all running events, competing in the most important and prestigious sports event – the Olympics – it would change world attitudes about women's capability. Everyone everywhere understands that 26.2 miles (or 42.2k) is a long way to run, and when they see women doing it they know that women can do anything and should be allowed to participate.

AL: Is there anything else to be done for women in sports?

KS: A lot yet needs to be done! There are many countries in the world where women are not allowed out of their houses alone, not allowed to drive cars, get an education or participate in sports. So getting the opportunities to these women will not be easy. We are working on ways to reach them, especially using technology and starting our new 261 running clubs (261 is my bib number from my first Boston Marathon and has come to mean 'fearless in the face of adversity'). We've only been going two and a half years but we're already in 11 countries and working with 5,000 women – every woman who has ever run has benefited from it and is more empowered as a result.

AL: And, when you run today, do you still think about that first finish line?

KS: Of course, I think about it all the time. But more than that, I think about that 20-year-old girl who had the courage to press on and finish – because it would have been so much easier to simply cover my face and walk off the course but I knew if I would do that I'd regret it. And I felt a responsibility to women. I knew that if I failed they'd all be told once again that women are always trying to go into places where they're not welcome and can't do it anyway. I proved that's not the case.

Your Chapter 10 Action Plan

- Pack your post-race bag

- Arrive at race

- Pick up bib

- Toilet stop

- Warm up

- Strip off (mostly)

- Toilet again

- START

- FINISH

- BE PROUD

Epilogue

When I set out to write this book I didn't expect to share both my heart as well as my soles. The brief was simple: write a book about going well far, but as I started to unpick my running journey I came to realise that my running life and personal life aren't mutually exclusive. I wouldn't have found my way with one if I hadn't experienced the other. And so, I parked any embarrassment I felt about admitting I had lost control of my 'healthy life' and *I Can Run* was born.

People will assure you they do not lose respect for others suffering from issues like I've experienced, but it's a hard bias to overcome. If my heartfelt account of how finding my feet in my late 20s has changed the course of the rest of my life can do anything to help you take the first steps to a happier, healthier life, then I'll be immensely pleased. The only question now is what are you waiting for?

'You know you are a runner when you automatically see 10k as 6.2 miles not £10,000'

Training Plans

Whether you're just buying your first trainers or are an experienced 5k'er looking to go further, starting a plan if you've never done one before is tough. First off, there's the structure (a bit like your colour-coded school timetable that invariably gave you a headache) and then there's the time commitments and confusing language.

So, before diving headfirst into a demanding training schedule, ask yourself these questions:
- What is my current fitness level?
- How much time do I have to train?
- How much time do I have for recovery?
- Would I be happy just to finish a race?
- Will I be happy doing all my exercise solo?

Have these answers to hand when looking for your training plan. In an ideal world, every runner would have a unique plan but that's not realistic. And so I have shared the training advice handed to me by my running coaches past and present.

(Oh, and as a heads-up . . . Don't stress too much about the exactness of the 400m or 200m suggestions – or the fact that you're switching between metres and miles – for the sprint sessions to come. They are presented like this because the best place to do them is on a track, which are 400m per lap. If you're not near one, going to the local park and guestimating a circuit will work equally well.)

STARTING A REGULAR RUNNING ROUTINE

Your coach: Anthony Fletcher, Onetrack
For true beginners you'll be pleased to know that your week should look relatively uneventful. The focus is increasing time on feet relative to time spent on the sofa. Go and find a flat bit of park and start with interval training.

Here's an example session:
• 1 minute of running
• 1 minute of walking
• Repeat 10 times

That's a 20-minute workout. Try and do this two more times in a week. But keep the intensity low.

Not yet up to 1 minute of running? Embrace the run/walk technique. The NHS Couch to 5K app will help you gradually work towards running 5k in 9 weeks. The plan involves 3 runs a week, with a day of rest in between, and a different schedule for each week. Available on iOS and Android.

RUNNING YOUR FIRST SUB-2HR HALF MARATHON

Your coach: Track Life LDN
This sample half-marathon plan will get you up to speed on
13.1 – but only if you follow the structure and put in the hours
in the gym too (see chapter 5).

TYPES OF RUNS + PACES ON THE PLAN

Race pace: for sub-2hr half marathon you need to run faster
than 9.09min/hr or faster per mile.

Easy run
Easy runs should be done 30 seconds to 1 minute per mile
slower than your half-marathon goal pace.

Long run
This is a long, slow distance run that will build your endurance.
Run at an easy pace; you should be able to hold a conversation.
This should be 30 seconds to 1 minute per mile slower than
your goal pace, too.

Intervals
In your shorter, faster intervals focus on good running form
and working at a higher intensity than your HM (half-marathon)
pace.

Tempo

This is a run holding the pace that you hope to maintain in the race. Remember, for sub-2hr you need to run faster than 9.09min/m.

COACH'S TIPS:

Listen to your body

Muscle soreness is expected with harder runs, but recognise the difference between pain and soreness. If you feel pain lingering, go and get a professional opinion instead of running through it. Hard workouts take up to two days to recover from.

Gradually build up

It's tempting to hit the miles fast and hard as you begin your plan, but remember the first few weeks are aimed at building a foundation. Ease yourself in and play for the long game, as it's consistency that will get you that PB!

Enjoy it

Some people love to run with others, some love running around attractive scenery, some like treadmills. Find what works best for you. If you enjoy your training you are more likely to stick to your plan!

	Monday REST	Tuesday INTERVALS/EASY RUN	Wednesday CROSS-TRAIN	Thursday TEMPO PACE AND HILLS	Friday GYM STRENGTH	Saturday REST	Sunday LONG RUN
1		3 miles easy		2 miles easy, 5 x 45 seconds hills @75% effort with jog/walk down recovery, 2 miles easy			6 miles
2		1 mile warm up 10 x 200m @75% effort with 60 seconds recovery, 1 mile warm down		1 mile easy, 3 x 1 mile @ HM pace with 90 seconds recovery, 1 mile easy			7 miles
3		4 miles easy		2 miles easy, 6 x 45 seconds hills @75% effort with jog/walk down recovery, 2 miles easy			8 miles
4		1 mile warm up 6 x 400m @75% effort with 90 seconds recovery, 1 mile warm down		1 mile easy, 4 x 1 mile @ HM pace with 90 seconds recovery, 1 mile easy			5 miles

5		5 miles easy		2 miles easy, 5 x 60 seconds hills @75% effort with jog/ walk down recovery, 2 miles easy			9 miles
6		1 mile warm up, 12 x 200m effort with 60 seconds recovery, 1 mile warm down		1 mile easy, 5 x 1 mile @ HM pace with 90 seconds recovery, 1 mile easy			10 miles
7		6 miles easy		2 miles easy, 6 x 60 seconds hills @75% effort with jog/ walk down recovery, 2 miles easy			11 miles
8		1 mile warm up, 8 x 400m with 90 - seconds recovery, 1 mile warm down		1 mile easy, 2 x 2 miles @ HM pace with 90 seconds recovery, 1mile easy			5 miles
9		7 miles easy		1 mile easy, 3 miles @ HM pace, 1 mile easy			12 miles
10		1 mile warm up 14 x 200m with 60 seconds recovery 1 mile warm down		1 mile easy, 3 x 2 miles @ HM pace with 90 seconds recovery, 1mile easy			13 miles

| 11 | | 5 miles easy | | 1 mile easy, 4 miles @ HM pace, 1 mile easy | | | 6 miles |
| 12 | rest | 3 miles easy and 10x 100m strides @ HM pace | rest or x train | 3 miles easy | rest | rest | race day |

RUNNING YOUR FIRST SUB 4-HR MARATHON

Your coach: Track Life LDN

I've run marathons for the joy that's in it and I've run races to beat the clock. For the latter, this is the plan I followed.

TYPES OF RUNS + PACES ON THE PLAN

Race pace

For a 4hr marathon you need to run a 9.09min/m. I trained for the target time of 3hr 55mins, or an 8:58 min/m so sub-4hr.

Easy run

Easy runs should be done 30 seconds to 1 minute per mile slower than marathon goal pace, e.g. 9:40–10:05 min/m.

Long run

This is a long, slow run that will build your endurance and get you used to long distances. Run at an easier pace. This should be slower than your marathon pace, e.g. 9:30–9:45min/m.

Intervals

In your shorter, faster intervals focus on good running form and working at a higher intensity than your marathon pace. These are here to get you used to a higher turnover of your feet and to increase your lactate threshold.

Threshold pace

This is faster than your marathon pace – it should be challenging but not so tough that you can't sustain the speed over a distance. For your marathon goal you should be aiming for a 8:15–8:35 min/m threshold pace.

PLAN STRUCTURE

This plan was designed around my week. I was already running regularly before starting it. Tip: if your week isn't set up for a long run on a Saturday then don't try to follow in my footsteps exactly. Instead, start the plan on the day that makes most sense for your long run to fall.

Week / weekly mileage	Monday TRACK INTERVAL PACE	Tuesday REST	Wednesday EASY/STEADY PACE	Thursday TEMPO/ THRESHOLD PACE	Friday REST	Saturday LONG RUN	Sunday REST
1 (25 miles)	1 mile @9:45 pace, 6 x 800m (goal time 3:39 for 800m) with 90 seconds recovery, 1 mile @9:45 pace		5 miles @9:30 pace	5 miles @8:33 pace		12 miles @9:43 pace	
2 (29 miles)	1 mile @9:45 pace, 5 x 1000m (goal time 4:37 for 1000m) with 2 mins recovery, 1 mile @9:45 pace		6 miles @9:30 pace	1 mile @9:30 3 miles @8:13 1 mile @9:30 pace		13 miles @9:43 pace	
3 (31 miles)	1 mile @9:45 pace, 3 x 1600m (goal time 7:37 for 1000m) with 90 seconds recovery, 1 mile @9:45 pace		7 miles @9:30 pace	5 miles @8:23 pace		14 miles @9:43 pace	

Week / weekly mileage	Monday TRACK INTERVAL PACE	Tuesday REST	Wednesday EASY/STEADY PACE	Thursday TEMPO/ THRESHOLD PACE	Friday REST	Saturday LONG RUN	Sunday REST
4 (29 miles)	1 mile @9:45 pace, 2 x 1200m (goal time 5:36 for 1200m) with 2 mins recovery 4 x 800m (goal time 3:39 for 800m) with 90 seconds recovery 1 mile @9:45 pace		8 miles @9:30 pace	7 miles @8:33 pace		8 miles @9:43 pace	
5 (30 miles)	1 mile @9:45 pace, 12 x 400m (goal time 1:46 for 400m) with 75 seconds recovery, 1 mile @9:45 pace		5 miles @9:30 pace	5 miles @8:23 pace		15 miles @9:43 pace	
6 (32 miles)	1 mile @9:45 pace, 6 x 800m (goal time 3:39 for 800m) with 80 seconds recovery, 1 mile @9:45 pace		6 miles @9:30 pace	1 mile @9:30 3 mile @8:13 1 mile @9:30		16 miles @9:43 pace	

Week / weekly mileage	Monday TRACK INTERVAL PACE	Tuesday REST	Wednesday EASY/STEADY PACE	Thursday TEMPO/ THRESHOLD PACE	Friday REST	Saturday LONG RUN	Sunday REST
7 (39 miles)	1 mile @9:45 pace, 6 x 1000m (goal time 4:37 for 1000m) with 2 mins recovery, 1 mile @9:45 pace		7 miles @9:30 pace	10 miles @8:58 pace		17 miles @9:43 pace	
8 (28 miles)	1 mile @9:45 pace, 4 x 1600m (goal time 7:37 for 1600m) with 90 seconds recovery, 1 mile @9:45 pace		8 miles @9:30 pace	5 miles @8:23 pace		9 miles @9:43 pace	
9 (39 miles)	1 mile @9:45 pace, 2 x 1200m (goal time 5:36 for 1200m) with 2 mins recovery 5 x 800m (goal time 3:39 for 800m) 1 mile @9:45 pace off 90 seconds recovery		5 miles @9:30 pace	10 miles @8:58 pace		18 miles @9:43 pace	

Week / weekly mileage	Monday TRACK INTERVAL PACE	Tuesday REST	Wednesday EASY/STEADY PACE	Thursday TEMPO/ THRESHOLD PACE	Friday REST	Saturday LONG RUN	Sunday REST
10 (37 miles)	1 mile @9:45 pace, 14 x 400m (goal time 1:46 for 400m) with 75 seconds recovery, 1 mile @9:45 pace		6 miles @9:30 pace	5 miles @8:23 pace		20 miles @9:33 pace	
11 (34 miles)	1 mile @9:45 pace, 2 sets of: 1 x 2000m (goal time 9:34) with 2 mins recovery 1 x 1200m (goal time 5:36) with 90 seconds recovery 1 x 800m (goal time 3:39) With 75 seconds recovery, 1 x 400m (goal time 1:46) (400m easy jog between sets) 1 mile @9:45 pace		7 miles @9:30 pace	10 miles @8:58 pace		12 miles @8:58 pace	

Week / weekly mileage	Monday TRACK INTERVAL PACE	Tuesday REST	Wednesday EASY/STEADY PACE	Thursday TEMPO/ THRESHOLD PACE	Friday REST	Saturday LONG RUN	Sunday REST
12 (42 miles)	1 mile @9:45 pace, 3 x 2000m (goal time 2000m 9:34) with 3 mins recovery 1 mile @9:45 pace		8 miles @9:30 pace	8 miles @8:58 pace		20 miles @9:20 pace	
13 (29 miles)	1 mile @9:45 pace, 1 x 1600m (goal time 7:37) 1 x 3200 (goal time 15:46) 2 x 800m (goal time 3.39 per 800m) 2 mins recovery, between every rep 1 mile @9:45 pace		7 miles @9:30 pace	5 miles @8:23 pace		12 miles @8:58 pace	
14 (23 miles)	1 mile @9:45 pace, 15 x 200m (goal time 50 seconds per 200m) with 45 seconds recovery, 1 mile @9:45 pace		5 miles @9:30 pace	2 miles @9:30 3 mile @8:13 1 mile @9:30 pace		8 miles @8:58 pace	

Week / weekly mileage	Monday TRACK INTERVAL PACE	Tuesday REST	Wednesday EASY/STEADY PACE	Thursday TEMPO/ THRESHOLD PACE	Friday REST	Saturday LONG RUN	Sunday REST
15 30(ish) miles	1 mile @9:45 pace, 8 x 200m (goal time 50 secs per 200m) 30 seconds recovery, 1 mile @9:45 pace	TOTAL REST	Easy 20/30 min run and stretch	3 miles @8:58	Easy 20 min shake out and stretch	TOTAL REST	RACE DAY

Your Little Black Book Of Running

If *I Can Run* has made you hungry for more, use my LBB to satisfy your cravings. This guide will help you bypass questionable fitness sources flying around social media, and instead go straight to the resources that have helped thousands run – and become – their best.

Expert Advice

Anita Bean

Anita is an award-winning registered nutritionist, health writer, internationally published author and champion athlete. She is accredited by the Association for Nutrition (AfN) and specialises in sport and exercise nutrition. Anita regularly debunks the myths surrounding a vegetarian diet and covers popular topics such as what to eat before and after exercise, how much protein you need and which supplements actually work.
@anitabean1; anitabean.co.uk

Georgie Bruinvels

Elite runner, exercise physiologist and research scientist Dr Georgie Bruinvels works with athletes and sportswomen to help them understand how hormone changes during the menstrual cycle impact all elements of training and performance, including

general wellness, metabolism, biomechanics and training adaptation. She studied for her PhD at University College London, looking at iron metabolism in endurance athletes with a specific focus on the menstrual cycle, and today is the driving force of the @fitrwoman project – an app that puts maximising your menstrual cycle into the palm of your hands.
@fitrwoman; fitrwoman.com

Andrew Cohen-Wray

Andrew Cohen-Wray, an athlete with over two and a half decades of competitive experience, helps people of any sporting ability achieve the same mindset used by top-level athletes. His goal is simple: to offer the same level of service that Olympic-grade athletes receive to the everyday athlete.
@athleteinmind; athleteinmind.co.uk

Anthony Fletcher

Anthony Fletcher is a personal trainer specialising in biomechanics. He is the founder of Onetrack run club and works with elite runners and everyday athletes alike, coaching regular gym-goers and Olympic hopefuls. He offers remote coaching or weekly track sessions in London. Whatever goal you're chasing, he can help you get there.
@aka_fletch; anthony-fletcher.com

David Hastie

With his experience as a competitive athlete and understanding of sports injury, David knows how to safely get the best out of his clients. His approach combines training with rehab when required. I trained with him in 2018 and his expertise helped me home in on my weaknesses – and fix them!
@twentytwotraining; twentytwotraining.com

Rory Knight

Rory is an elite fitness expert, Global Master Trainer for Technogym and celebrated coach who can help you reach peak fitness without losing your personality; his training techniques are science-backed but delivered with a unique style of motivation. As co-creator of @track_life_ldn he's helping to make training like an athlete accessible to all.
@roryknightfitness; tracklifeldn.com

Camilla Langlands

Camilla is a London Marathon pacer who has run more than 148 marathons, and 100 of those have been with her mother Jacquie Millett. It's safe to say that what she doesn't know about race-day prep (probably) isn't worth knowing.
@thisishowwerun_ ; thisishowwerun.com

Omar Mansour

As a coach who has trained under Great Britain coaches (Omar is an 800m athlete himself) Mr OMG, as he's known on social media, fuses personal experience with professional qualifications. This makes him both knowledgeable and empathetic to a runner's needs. Join him with his co-conspirator Rory Knight at Track Life LDN training sessions.
@mromg; tracklifeldn.com

Emma Kirk Odunubi

Emma is a running biomechanics nerd who matches the perfect footwear to the individual runner, and takes pride in being known as the trainer geek. Follow her social posts of easy-to-digest trainer talk.
@emmakirkyo; emmakirkodunubi.co.uk

Bradley Scanes

Brad Scanes is a specialist musculoskeletal physiotherapist who works with footballers, Team GB gymnasts and clients like you or me to prevent and overcome injuries. An avid runner himself, Brad knows how to avoid the common pitfalls of going well far; he shaved 42 minutes off his marathon time by nailing the perfect plan.

@physiobrad; physiobrad.co.uk

Joslyn Thompson Rule

Joslyn has 17 years' experience as a Personal Trainer and Sports Therapist. Studying and teaching health and wellness 'rocks her world'! She is passionate about training smarter not harder, which is why she was handpicked by Nike as one of their Global Master Trainers 10 years ago. When not coaching you'll find her competing in CrossFit, having formerly competed in rowing, marathons, triathlons and kettlebell sport. The demands of this sport have led to an obsession with recovery; a former coach once taught her that 'you work (recover) to play (train/compete)'.

@joslynthompsonrule; joslynthompsonrule.com

Luke Worthington

Personal trainer, coach and industry educator Luke Worthington has a lifetime of experience in international and elite level sport. Outside the gym he runs international strength training seminars and mentors young trainers through the Nike Academy. He's a strong force for change in the industry and is passionate about training well, not more.

he Brititsh sprint sensation gives you a AAA pass to athlete
life along with unfiltered commentary on her days out of spikes.

Susie Chan
@susie_chan
Sometimes 26.2 just isn't enough, so follow endurance runner
Susie Chan for ultra inspiration. Follow her runcations around
the world and be pepped up by her sunny personality.

Jacky Hunt-Broersma
@ncrunnerjacky
Jacky lost her leg to cancer, but rather than that be the end of
her running journey, it was the start of a new one. Jacky has
built up a good portfolio of firsts for female amputees in trail
running, proving the naysayers wrong and building a path for
other amputee runners. Her favourite running distance is 50
miles. She's also a mum and her young daughter will often run
with her.

Brigid Kosgei
@brigidkosgei
In 2019 Brigid Kosegi beat Paula Radcliffe's 16-year marathon
record. She's now the women's marathon world record holder
– if that's not a reason to follow her then you've probably just
read the wrong book.

83*

Morgan Mitchell

@morganmitch

As courageous off the track and she is on it, Aussie vegan runner Morgan Mitchell is the runner you may not be following, but need too. I have a serious girl crush.

Paula Radcliffe

@Paula_radcliffe

Just because she's hung up her professional kit doesn't mean Radcliffe has stopped running. No. The three-time London Marathon winner now uses her sporting profile to keep the conversation about running alive. Follow for updates from one of the greats of modern athletics.

Volt Women

@voltwomen

This global platform pushes race times and women's agendas. Follow to be part of a global discussion and community.

BEDTIME READING

Books that I've read and that have impacted my life in and out of Lycra:

Anita Bean: *Vegetarian Meals in 30 Minutes: More than 100 Delicious Recipes for Fitness* (Bloomsbury Sport, 2019)

Natasha Devon: *A Beginner's Guide to Being Mental: An A–Z from Anxiety to Zero F**ks Given* (Bluebird, 2018)

Bryony Gordon: *Eat, Drink, Run: How I Got Fit Without Going Too Mad* (Headline, 2018)

Phil Knight: *Shoe Dog: A Memoir by the Creator of NIKE* (Simon & Schuster UK, 2018)

Sarah Knight: *The Life-Changing Magic of Not Giving a F**k* (Quercus, 2015)

Christopher McDougall: *Born to Run: The Hidden Tribe, the Ultra-Runners and the Greatest Race the World Has Never Seen* (Profile Books, 2010)

Christopher McDougall: *Running with Sherman: The Donkey Who Survived Against All Odds and Raced Like a Champion* (Profile Books, 2019)

Ella Mills: *Deliciously Ella: The Plant-Based Cookbook* (Yellow Kite, 2018)

Haruki Murakami: *What I Talk About When I Talk About Running* (Vintage, 2009)

Jody Shield: *Self-Care for the Soul: Power Up Your Brightest, Boldest, Happiest You* (Yellow Kite, 2019)

Handy Apps

Aaptiv

The running coach you wish you had but don't! With a library of treadmill sessions to choose from, this audio workout helps make light work of speedwork.

Audible

For all the books I want to read but don't have the time to there's Audible. This app became my trusty running buddy when marathon training.

Couch to 5K

From your first minute to your first mile and beyond. There's a reason that this is one of the most successful fitness apps of the decade – it works.

FitrWoman

This app helps you plan your miles around your menstrual cycle for peak performance. It also has nutrition help and is used by professional sportswomen. Download, pronto.

My Pollen Forecast UK

As an allergy-induced asthma sufferer I don't look forward to spring, nor summer for that matter – 'tis the season of streaming eyes, a snotty nose and running with an inhaler. But knowing when the pollen count is going to rise helps me manage my allergy and asthma difficulties (read: I run indoors).

MapMyRun

Use to track your runs and then analyse your data. Personally I find their online version better than their app – I use this to plan new routes in London but also when I travel for work around the world.

Pace Converter

The handiest app of them all. Use to figure out your min/km or km/h for treadmill sessions and also race pace.

Strava

Use to find routes and running buddies, along with using Strava Beacon on the iOS app to share your real-time location with family and friends. There are few things that this app can't do – apart from actually doing the run for you.

USEFUL WEBSITES

261® Fearless

261fearless.org

Find like-minded active women who encourage a positive sense of self and fearlessness in each other. Essentially, come together and unleash your inner Switzer.

Find a Race

findarace.com

Their motto is 'finding a challenge is no longer challenging' – you get the gist.

Mind – Food and Mood

mind.org.uk

This site provides useful insights exploring the relationship between what you eat and how you feel.

New Scientist

newscientist.com

For all the really nerdy research stuff that can keep you up to speed with the world of health.

Run Britain

runbritain.com

The best race info and training advice for UK road runners.

Outside Online

outsideonline.com

Interesting reads and advice on active, adventurous lifestyles from across the pond.

Runner's World

runnersworld.co.uk

Tips, trainer reviews and interviews with some of the brightest minds in running.

Tempo

tempojournal.com

Come here for profiles of people who just bloody love running. It's inspiration from Down Under.

Well + Good

wellandgood.com

A website devoted to healthy advice. Catch their running stories for reads that talk to you like your BFF.

USEFUL HELPLINES

Anorexia & Bulimia Care (ABC)

03000 11 12 13; anorexiabulimiacare.org.uk

ABC is a national UK eating disorders organisation with over 25 years' experience. Ongoing care, emotional support and practical guidance for anyone affected by eating disorders.

Beat

0808 801 0677; helplines are open Monday–Friday 12pm–8pm and weekends and bank holidays 4pm–8pm. You can also email the team at help@beateatingdisorders.org.uk; beateatingdisorders.org.uk

Beat is the UK's eating disorder charity. They are a champion, guide and friend to anyone affected by eating disorders, giving individuals experiencing an eating disorder and their loved ones a place where they feel listened to, supported and empowered.

CALM (Campaign Against Living Miserably)

0800 58 58 58 (5pm–midnight); thecalmzone.net
Provides listening services, information and support for men at risk of suicide, including webchat (5pm–midnight).

Mind

0300 123 3393 (lines are open 9am–6pm, Monday–Friday (except bank holidays); info@mind.org.uk
Provides information on a range of topics including: types of mental-health problems; where to get help; medication and alternative treatments and advocacy.

Samaritans

116 123 (freephone); samaritans.org
Freepost RSRB-KKBY-CYJK, PO Box 9090, Stirling FK8 2SA
24-hour emotional support for anyone struggling to cope.

SANEline

0300 304 7000 (4.30pm–10.30pm every day); sane.org.uk
Helpline offering practical information and emotional support in a crisis.

Acknowledgements

Back in 2018 I had a wild idea to start a running podcast. Not just any running podcast; one that included interviewing people while on a 5KM. "Well, that sounds interesting," said Hannah Russell, founder of podcast production agency Mags Creative. "Let's try it."

Since then, Hannah and her team have backed my fast-paced ideas and zest for breaking the rules to help me create Well Far: The Running Podcast. Without them, this book would still just be an item on my bucket list yet to be crossed off.

I'll always be grateful for their belief in me and for all the thousands of women who tuned into the podcast, including Yellow Kite's Editorial Director Lauren Whelan who, after listening to the show, took a chance on me and commissioned this book. She's helped me navigate the bumpy road of writing a book and what a journey it's been.

But, there's one person who's been there every single step of the way and that's my husband, Ted. More than just a shoulder to cry on or someone to vent to, Ted took on the lion's share of *I Can Run*. Helping with interviews, words and ideas. We sat together in our kitchen mind-mapping chapters and endlessly researching experts, then begging for their time to bring you the best of the best advice. And when not writing,

Ted joined me on runs to sweat test the advice in this book. He's a keeper.

Outside of the running and writing world the support for this project goes on for miles and miles. The constant WhatsApp messages from siblings, friends, family and industry pals helped keep me on track when, at times, all I wanted to do was run a million miles away from this manuscript. Baring your heart and soles isn't easy, but their enthusiasm to see the end result stopped me from hitting the wall and pushed me through any writing barriers.

And then there's my mum. My biggest cheerleader in life. As you'll know from the pages in this book, life hasn't been easy – far from it. But from a young age she taught me to be strong, to not give-up and to always look for sunshine on grey days – messages that I hope are evident in these pages.

My last shout out goes to you. Thank you for believing in yourself enough to buy the book and sticking with me through to the end. Here's to the next leg of our journeys.

Resources

INTRODUCTION

www.brookings.edu/opinions/are-children-raised-with-absent-
fathers-worse-off/
www.outdoorsradar.com/run/strava-run-commuting/
www.jospt.org/doi/full/10.2519/jospt.2014.5164
www.psychologytoday.com/us/blog/living-single/200901/
children-single-mothers-how-do-they-really-fare
www.standard.co.uk/lifestyle/health/what-is-burnout-how-to-
cope-a4154276.html

CHAPTER 1

www.schneiderelectricparismarathon.com/en/event/key-figures
www.runnersworld.com/uk/training/motivation/a773110/
qa-kathrine-switzer/
www.telegraph.co.uk/athletics/2019/04/28/london-marathon-
2019-charlotte-purdue-clocks-third-fastest-time/
www.runnersworld.com/runners-stories/a28787943/
overcoming-obstacles-brittany-runs-a-marathon/

www.ncbi.nlm.nih.gov/pubmed/28522092
www.npr.org/2011/03/28/134861448/put-those-shoes-on-
running-wont-kill-your-knees?t=1567088010405

CHAPTER 2

www.discovery.ucl.ac.uk/1399896/1/103.full.pdf
www.refinery29.com/en-gb/kathrine-switzer-interview
www.runnersworld.com/uk/training/motivation/
a26748147/a-history-of-womens-running/
www.journals.sagepub.com/doi/
full/10.1177/1474474013491927
www.sportengland.org/media/13768/active-lives-adult-may-17-
18-report.pdf
www.runnersworld.com/training/a20785273/why-are-runners-
often-called-harriers/
www.ukactive.com/wp-content/uploads/2019/03/ActiveLab_
Report_The_Current_State_Of_FitTech_Web.pdf
www.wareable.com/sport/strava-app-complete-guide-875

CHAPTER 3

www.sciencedaily.com/releases/2015/02/150203204451.htm
www.sah.org.ar/pdf/eritropatias/CADAE1408C.pdf
www.pennmedicine.org/updates/blogs/health-and-
wellness/2015/may/
are-women-athletes-more-susceptible-to-injury
www.runnersworld.com/uk/training/marathon/a27787958/
average-marathon-finish-time/

CHAPTER 4

www.womenshealthmag.com/uk/food/healthy-eating/a708471/
carbs-and-weight-loss/
www.healthline.com/nutrition/eat-after-workout#section7
www.bbc.co.uk/news/health-38562048
www.thebodycoach.com/blog/busting-the-myth-that-eating-
carbs-after-6pm-will-make-you-fat-40.html

CHAPTER 5

www.journals.lww.com/nsca-jscr/Abstract/2017/01000/The_
Effect_of_Strength_Training_on_Performance.2.aspx
www.salford.ac.uk/news/articles/2018/12million-runners-in-uk-
injured-new-research
www.greatist.com/fitness/why-all-runners-should-
strength-train
file:///Users/alane/Downloads/SN03336.pdf
www.ncbi.nlm.nih.gov/pmc/articles/PMC3290924/
www.greatist.com/fitness/why-all-runners-should-strength-
train#Exercises-All-Runners-Should-Do

CHAPTER 6

www.health.harvard.edu/staying-healthy/understanding-the-
stress-response
www.dnafit.com/advice/fitness/cortisol-stress-and-exercise.asp
www.psychologytoday.com/gb/blog/heart-and-soul-
healing/201303/dr-herbert-benson-s-relaxation-response
www.nhs.uk/news/pregnancy-and-child/study-fails-to-prove-
effects-of-stress-on-fertility/

CHAPTER 7

www.bbc.co.uk/news/stories-45561334
www.manrepeller.com/2018/07/on-again-off-again-relationship-advice.html

CHAPTER 8

www.bbc.co.uk/sport/athletics/30927245
www.bbc.co.uk/sport/48243310
www.rd.com/culture/moments-that-changed-womens-history/
www.aims-worldrunning.org/statistics.html
www.bbc.co.uk/news/world-49284389
www.theguardian.com/lifeandstyle/2018/sep/16/athlete-breastfed-son-during-ultra-marathon

References

INTRODUCTION

1   www.blog.strava.com/press/2018-year-in-sport

CHAPTER 1

2   www.runnerclick.com/marathon-finishing-times-study-and-
    statistics/
3   www.researchgate.net/journal/1531-5320_Psychonomic_Bulletin_
    Review
4   www.ncbi.nlm.nih.gov/pubmed/28365296
5   www.ncbi.nlm.nih.gov/pmc/articles/PMC3632802/
6   www.ncbi.nlm.nih.gov/pubmed/2360871
7   www.npr.org/2011/03/28/134861448/put-those-shoes-on-running-
    wont-kill-your-knees?t=1567088010405
8   www.ncbi.nlm.nih.gov/pubmed/9526893?ordinalpos=1&itool=En-
    trezSystem2.
    PEntrez.Pubmed.Pubmed_ResultsPanel.Pubmed_DiscoveryPanel.
    Pubmed_Discovery_RA&linkpos=1&log%24=relatedarticles&logd
    bfrom=pubmed
9   www.statista.com/statistics/934996/running-participation-uk

CHAPTER 2

10 www.apps.apple.com/gb/app/one-you-couch-to-5k/id1082307672
11 www.blog.strava.com/press/2018-year-in-sport/

12 www.ukactive.com/news/public-leisure-generates-over-3-3bn-in-social-value-to-the-uk/;www.sportengland.org/media/13768/active-lives-adult-may-17-18-report.pdf

CHAPTER 3
13 www.runnersconnect.net/excess-weight-and-running/
14 www.ncbi.nlm.nih.gov/pmc/articles/PMC4281377/

CHAPTER 4
15 www.beateatingdisorders.org.uk/media-centre/eating-disorder-statistics
16 www.womenshealthmag.com/uk
17 www.dove.com/us/en/stories/about-dove/our-research.html
18 www.ncbi.nlm.nih.gov/pubmed/29466592
19 www.ncbi.nlm.nih.gov/pubmed/26568522
20 www.mdpi.com/2072-6643/10/12/1841/htm
21 www.ncbi.nlm.nih.gov/pubmed/17490455

CHAPTER 5
22 www.sportengland.org/media/10083/insight_go-where-women-are.pdf
23 www.ncbi.nlm.nih.gov/pmc/articles/PMC3290924/
24 www.ncbi.nlm.nih.gov/pubmed/24532151

CHAPTER 6
25 www.nytimes.com/2008/03/02/sports/playmagazine/02play-physed.html

CHAPTER 7
26 www.ncbi.nlm.nih.gov/pmc/articles/PMC5932411

CHAPTER 8
27 www.fitrwoman.com/post/press-release-largest-global-studyof-active-women

28 www.fitrwoman.com/post/press-release-largest-global-studyof-active-women

29 www.fitrwoman.com/post/press-release-largest-global-studyof-active-women

CHAPTER 9

30 www.bbc.co.uk/mediacentre/latestnews/2018/loneliest-age-group-radio-4

31 www.co-operative.coop/campaigning/loneliness

32 www.news.illinois.edu/view/6367/204883

33 www.ncbi.nlm.nih.gov/pubmed/31445953

34 www.pnas.org/content/108/7/3017

35 www.thelancet.com/journals/lancet/article/PIIS0140-6736(18)30578-6/fulltext

36 www.ncbi.nlm.nih.gov/pmc/articles/PMC6542067/

37 www.nature.com/articles/npp2017148

38 www.ncbi.nlm.nih.gov/pmc/articles/PMC2817271/

39 www.ncbi.nlm.nih.gov/pmc/articles/PMC2077351/

40 www.researchgate.net/publication/311861136_A_study_on_level_of_physical_activity_depression_anxiety_and_stress_symptoms_among_adolescents